Surgical Management of Thyroid and Parathyroid Diseases

C. Gopalakrishnan Nair
Santhosh John Abraham
Editors

Surgical Management of Thyroid and Parathyroid Diseases

Springer

Editors
C. Gopalakrishnan Nair
Professor of Surgery
Endocrine Surgery Division
Amrita Institute of Medical Sciences
and Research Centre
Kochi, Kerala, India

Santhosh John Abraham
Department of Surgery
Lourdes Hospital
Kochi, Kerala, India

ISBN 978-981-97-3773-4 ISBN 978-981-97-3774-1 (eBook)
https://doi.org/10.1007/978-981-97-3774-1

This Springer imprint is published by the registered company Springer Nature Singapore Pte Ltd.
The registered company address is: 152 Beach Road, #21-01/04 Gateway East, Singapore 189721, Singapore

Preface

Ayurveda, the traditional medicine in India has a long history, and Sushruta, the renounced master surgery in Ancient India, elaborates reconstruction of nasal deformities and the removal of urinary bladder stones in his chronicle. However, there are no authentic references to thyroidectomy in traditional Indian medicine.

Modern medicine was introduced to India in the nineteenth century and the major centres were mostly in urban areas. There was a high prevalence of iodine deficiency diseases in many areas of India and large volume-goitres were usual. However, complicated operations like thyroidectomy were performed only in a few major urban hospitals. The practice of thyroidectomy was not standardised and partial or subtotal thyroidectomy was practised.

Professor (Dr) Sivapatham Vittal initiated the attempts to streamline the surgical management of thyroid disease in India.

S. Vittal, MS, FRCS(Ed), FRCS (Eng), FICS, FIMSA, FAIS, FTASc, FAES, DSc (Hon) (Fig. 1).

Professor Vittal received undergraduate and post-graduate training at the prestigious Madras Medical College. He was impressed by the complexities of the endocrine system and developed a keen interest during his post-graduate days. He moved to the UK after his post-graduation and was deeply influenced by Mr. Selwyn Taylor

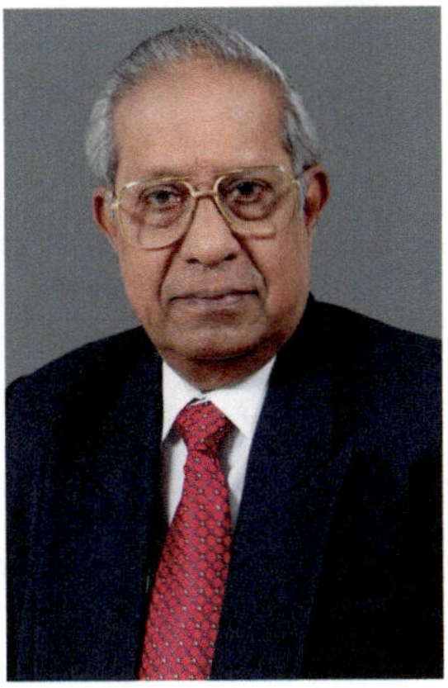

Fig. 1 Prof Sivapatham Vittal

and Professor R. B. Welbourn, acclaimed Endocrine Surgeons at Hammersmith Hospital, London, UK. He received the fellowship in Surgery from the Royal College of Surgeons of Edinburgh. He was awarded a Travelling Fellowship with Prof Ivan Johnston, a distinguished Endocrine Surgeon at Royal Victoria Infirmary at Newcastle-Upon-Tyne, UK.

Upon returning to India, he joined his alma mater as a faculty in the Department of Surgery. He was instrumental in creating the division of Endocrine Surgery in the Department of General Surgery at Madras Medical College and Government General Hospital, Chennai, in 1980, which culminated in a full-fledged Department of Endocrine Surgery in 1987, the first Department of Endocrine Surgery in India and South Asia (Fig. 2). He invited many Overseas Surgeons like Professor John Farndon, Professor Pady Boulter, and Mr Andrew Gunn to visit his department and organised many academic programmes to popularise Endocrine Surgery nationwide (Fig. 3).

He was instrumental in forming the Indian Association of Endocrine Surgeons in 1993, of which he was the Founder President. The organisation continues to be a prestigious platform for spreading knowledge in all aspects of endocrine surgery.

Professor Vittal is a widely appreciated teacher and was effective in spreading the message of safe thyroidectomy to budding surgeons. Because of its increasing prevalence, the knowledge and skill in managing thyroid diseases have to be disseminated to all practising surgeons and Professor Vittal plays a crucial role in this aspect.

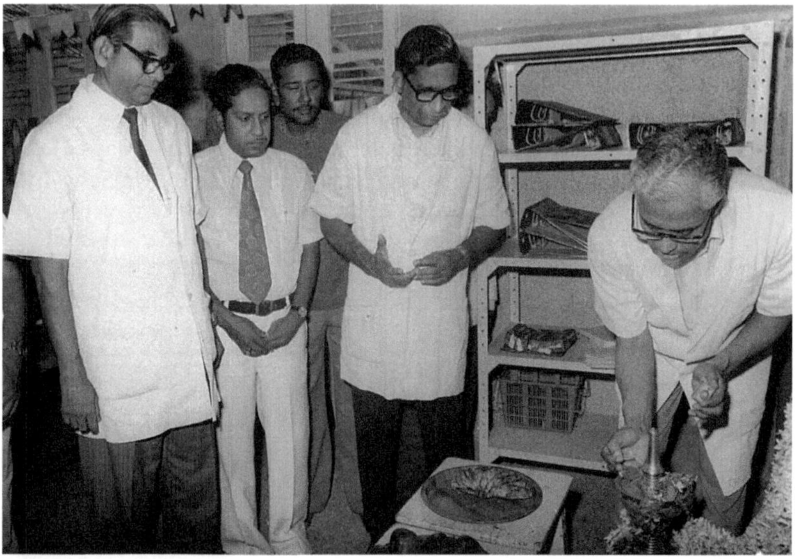

Fig. 2 Inauguration of Division of Endocrine Surgery in Madras Medical College & Government General Hospital, Chennai in 1980 which culminated in to the Department of Endocrine Surgery in 1987 - First in India and South Asia

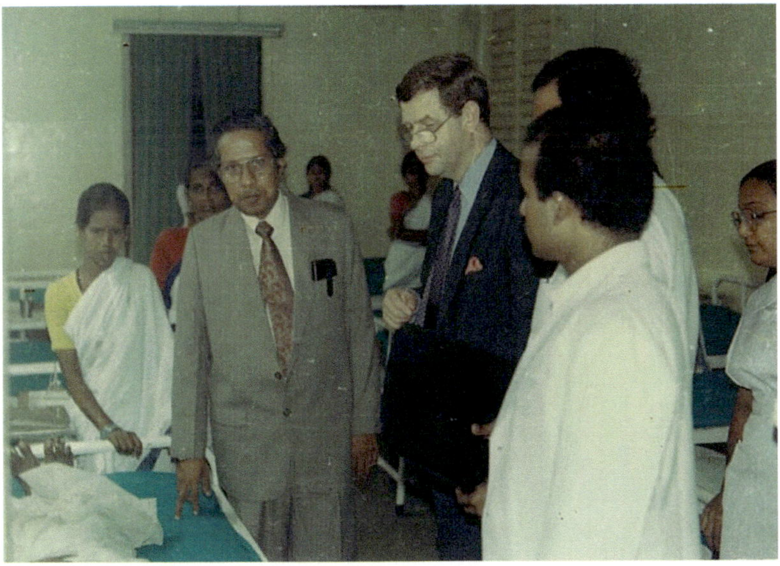

Fig. 3 Prof John Farndon with Prof S Vittal during his visit to Department of Endocrine Surgery in Madras Medical College & Government General Hospital, Chennai

He has been an eminent teacher for over 55 years, editing and publishing a *Surgical Endocrinology* book. He has been on the Editorial Board of several prestigious journals: the British Journal of Surgery, the World Journal of Endocrine Surgery, and the Indian Journal of Surgery.

Professor S Vittal is a recipient of the prestigious "Dr B C Roy National Award" for the year 1995 for developing the speciality of Surgical Endocrinology in India. This is the highest award given to a doctor by the Medical Council of India. In 2011, the Government of India awarded him the prestigious Padma Shri award, one of the highest civilian awards, for his yeoman service in Medicine.

For all his great contributions, he is popularly known as the "Father of Endocrine Surgery" in India.

Kochi, Kerala, India C. Gopalakrishnan Nair
Kochi, Kerala, India Santhosh John Abraham

Contents

1.3 Iodine Deficiency

Iodine is an essential nutrient that is not synthesised in our body. Hence, if it is unavailable in the diet, it leads to iodine deficiency. Iodine is essential for the thyroid hormone synthesis. Iodine deficiency disorders have been recognised as a significant health problem in India since 1962. In early childhood, it causes cognitive impairment and growth impairment. In adults, iodine deficiency causes goitre and hypothyroidism. However, mild to moderate inadequacy of iodine, the euthyroid state is maintained by excessive stimulation of the thyroid, resulting in an adenoma. Iodine replacement in the form of iodised salt decreases this risk. The goitre prevalence decreased considerably from 23% in 2003 to 15% in 2012, following the implementation of the universal salt iodisation programme [4]. Optimisation of iodine intake is essential in the prevention of thyroid disorders [5].

1.4 Hyperthyroidism

Hyperthyroidism is less frequent in the community compared to hypothyroidism and is characterised by weight loss, increased appetite, anxiety, restlessness, irritability, palpitations, bone pain and heat intolerance. Thyrotoxicosis is the clinical syndrome of excess thyroid hormone, irrespective of the source [6]. But, hyperthyroidism refers to thyrotoxicosis when the source of excess hormone is exaggerated synthesis in the thyroid gland. The most common causes of hyperthyroidism are diffuse toxic goitre (Graves' disease), toxic nodular goitre (Plummer's disease) and nodular toxic goitre or toxic thyroid adenoma. Iatrogenic thyrotoxicosis is not rare and occurs when the patient consumes an excess amount of the hormone. Thyrotoxicosis can also be due to a leak of thyroid hormones from the thyroid gland secondary to subacute thyroiditis. The laboratory studies are characterised by low serum TSH (sometimes <0.00 uIU/mL) with high T3 and T4 levels (Table 1.2).

The treatment options for hyperthyroidism include anti-thyroid drugs, radioactive iodine and thyroidectomy. The selection of treatment schedule is individualised based on clinical and imaging characteristics. Total thyroidectomy is an effective and relatively safe option and offers a permanent cure with acceptable morbidity in the hands of an experienced surgeon [7]. Thyroidectomy is relatively safe when the preoperative euthyroid status is achieved, and the refinement of surgical techniques and advanced energy sources for control of bleeding has reduced rates of complications like recurrent laryngeal nerve injury and hypoparathyroidism. After total thyroidectomy, post-operative hypothyroidism is expected and needs levothyroxine replacement therapy.

Table 1.2 Hyperthyroidism

Parameters	Levels	Normal range
TSH	Low	0.4–4.2 uIu/mL
Total T3	High	75–195 ng/dL
Total T4	High	4.6–11.2 mcg/dL

Table 1.3 Subclinical thyroid disorder

Diagnosis	Serum T3, T4	Serum TSH
Sub-clinical hypothyroidism	Normal	High
Sub-clinical hyperthyroidism	Normal	Low

Table 1.4 Interpretation of thyroid function tests

		TSH	TSH	TSH
		Low	Normal	High
T4	Low	Central hypothyroidism, non-thyroidal illness	Central hypothyroidism	Primary hypothyroidism
T4	Normal	Subclinical hyperthyroidism	Normal thyroid	Subclinical hypothyroidism
T4	High	Primary hyperthyroidism	TSH producing adenoma, thyroid hormone resistance	TSH producing adenoma, thyroid hormone resistance

Note: Besides the information in the table above, non-thyroidal illness (see text below) can cause unclassifiable thyroid function test results

1.5 Subclinical Thyroid Disease

Subclinical thyroid diseases include subclinical hypothyroidism and subclinical hyperthyroidism (Table 1.3), characterised by borderline thyroid dysfunction with subtle symptoms and diagnosed in laboratory studies (Table 1.4). Unless there are compelling indications to treat, treatment is not generally required. However, in certain situations, such as pregnancy, subclinical hypothyroidism requires active management.

1.6 Thyroiditis

Inflammation of the thyroid gland could be due to viral infection or autoimmunity, in which case the symptoms of thyrotoxicosis can occur due to the leaking of thyroid hormones. This illness commonly follows a viral infection and manifests as pain in the throat, difficulty swallowing, swelling in the neck, and relapsing fever, primarily not responding to anti-inflammatory drugs like acetaminophen in addition to clinical features of thyrotoxicosis like palpitations, weight loss and anxiety. A Technetium99 thyroid uptake scan will help to differentiate thyroiditis from Grave's disease. Radiopharmaceutical fails to concentrate in the thyroid gland in thyroiditis, whereas, in the latter, there is an increased uptake of radioactive iodine (Table 1.5). Treatment of thyroiditis involves only medical management with steroids and beta-blockers to decrease the palpitations. Some instances of thyroiditis may require surgery owing to a large volume thyroid swelling with pressure effects.

Table 1.5 Thyroiditis

Parameter	Graves' disease	Thyroiditis
Serum T3	High	High
Serum T4	High	High
Serum TSH	Low	Low
Antibodies (TSH R-Ab)[a]	Present	Absent
Thyroid radioactive iodine uptake scan	High uptake	Low uptake

[a] *TSH R-Ab* thyroid-stimulating hormone receptor antibody

1.7 Goitre

Goitre, which refers to thyroid swelling, can be diffuse or nodular. Goitres may be associated with thyroid hormonal dysfunction and, when associated with hypothyroidism, are treated medically. However, large goitres and associated pressure symptoms like difficulty in swallowing, cough or shortness of breath are treated surgically with total thyroidectomy.

Toxic nodular goitre is generally treated surgically after control of hyperthyroidism with anti-thyroid drugs. Routine evaluation of thyroid nodules, like ultrasound imaging and targeted cytology for characterisation of the nodules, are always done to exclude the possibility of malignancy. Recurrent thyroid cysts are rare, but thyroidectomy offers a permanent cure.

1.8 Thyroid Cancer

The thyroid gland develops cancers with different biological behaviours and is three times more common in women than in men [8]. The commonest thyroid cancer is differentiated thyroid cancer and has relatively slow progression and favourable outcomes. Papillary thyroid carcinoma constitutes up to 85% of thyroid cancers and is diagnosed by cytological studies of thyroid nodules. Medullary thyroid cancer arises from the parafollicular cells. The acceptable management regimen for differentiated thyroid cancer is thyroidectomy followed by radioiodine treatment and TSH suppression.

Several studies have identified the risk factors for a poor prognosis in thyroid cancers like age >45, male gender, familial disease, size >4 cm, multifocal disease, bilateral disease, extrathyroidal extension and distant metastases. Total thyroidectomy, which was the routine surgical practice for all thyroid cancers, is now recommended selectively based on clinical and tumour characteristics noted above.

The 10-year recurrence rate for differentiated thyroid carcinomas after total thyroidectomy is 7.7% compared to 9.8% after lobectomy [9].

Medullary carcinoma of the thyroid can be a sporadic cancer or component of MEN 2 syndrome ((Multiple Endocrine Neoplasia type 2). The only effective treatment is early surgery since adjuvant treatments are less effective.

1.9 Non-thyroidal Illness (NTI)

Non-thyroidal illness is also called sick euthyroid syndrome and occurs in acute illness, starvation and ICU patients. Abnormal thyroid hormone levels characterise NTI without intrinsic thyroid dysfunction. It may be associated with tissue-level hypothyroidism, which is not clinically evident because of the brief duration, as a protective response and should not be treated in general [10]. Notably, almost all types of unclassifiable thyroid function reports can coexist with NTI.

1.10 Pediatric Thyroid Disease and Surgery

Thyroid disease in paediatrics practice is less frequent and encompasses diverse benign and malignant conditions. Benign conditions include Graves' disease, toxic adenoma and goitre. Papillary thyroid cancers are occasionally seen in children, but after uncovering the genetics of medullary thyroid cancers in multiple endocrine neoplasia, prophylactic thyroidectomy gained significant interest. Since the ratio between tumour size and thyroid volume differs in children, conservative surgery, less than total removal, is not always recommended.

Near-total or total thyroidectomy with or without central lymph node dissection is the treatment of choice in thyroid cancer patients. The chances of complications following thyroidectomy are high in children, so surgery is better performed in a high-volume centre with an experienced surgeon [11]. However, these complication rates may be minimised in expert hands.

1.10.1 Congenital Hypothyroidism

Congenital hypothyroidism (CH) is one of the crucial causes of preventable mental retardation. It is caused in 85% of cases due to sporadic abnormal thyroid gland development called thyroid dysgenesis. The remaining 25% of congenital hypothyroidism is due to dyshormonogenesis. The symptoms of CH are subtle. Hence neonatal screening between days 2 to 5 should be done to avoid delayed diagnosis and consequent severe outcomes of CH like mental retardation. Once the diagnosis is made, thyroid hormone supplementation (levothyroxine initial dose, as per American Academy of Paediatrics and European Society of Pediatric Endocrinology, is 10–15 ugm/kg/day) achieves normalisation of thyroid hormone levels in 2 weeks and TSH returns to normal levels in 4 weeks [12].

1.10.2 Consumptive Hypothyroidism

Consumptive hypothyroidism is a rare and recently recognised clinical condition that occurs as a complication of Infantile hepatic haemangioma (IHH) due to increased synthesis of type 3 deiodinase enzyme by the tumour tissue. The altered enzyme degrades both T4 and T3 into the inactive reverse T3, and when this deactivation of thyroid hormones exceeds the synthesis, it results in hypothyroidism. Definitive treatment of the haemangioma and debulking the tumour tissue resolves this hypothyroidism [13].

1.10.3 Juvenile Autoimmune Hypothyroidism

The autoimmune process targeting the thyroid gland leads to euthyroid goitre, hypothyroidism and hyperthyroidism. Juvenile hypothyroidism (JH) adversely affects the growth, pubertal development and scholastic performance of children [14]. A study done in Eastern India on 100 subjects with less than 18 years of hypothyroidism showed that 74% were found to have overt hypothyroidism (OH), while only 26% had subclinical hypothyroidism (SCH). A family history of thyroid disorder in the family, with or without goitre, was present in a significant proportion of patients. There were higher female preponderance and Thyroid peroxidase antibody positivity with OH. The typical presentation includes goitre, weight gain, height deceleration and fatigue. The prevalence of short stature was higher in OH when compared to SCH. The treatment of juvenile autoimmune hypothyroidism is by thyroxine replacement, just like other causes of hypothyroidism, unless there are compression symptoms secondary to huge goitre, in which case, surgery is required in addition to the hormone replacement.

1.10.4 Hypothyroidism and Puberty

In general, children with hypothyroidism are associated with delayed sexual maturation and delayed puberty. However, there are exceptions when they may be associated precocious puberty [15].

1.10.5 Hyperthyroidism in Children

More than 90% of thyrotoxicosis in paediatric age group is attributed by Graves' disease. Anti-thyroid drugs (ATD) are the best initial treatment for paediatric age group. Major problem is the high relapse rate, up to 70%, however prolonged ATD therapy can result in 88% remission rate. In paediatric patients aged 5 years or younger with very large goitre, severe ophthalmopathy, persistent hyperthyroidism, unable to tolerate ATD due to side effects or not responding to ATD, it is advisable to undergo near total or total thyroidectomy [16].

1.10.6 Thyroid Nodules in Children

Thyroid toxic adenoma or 'hot' nodule is a benign condition that requires surgery, especially in paediatric population. Toxic adenomas are autonomously functioning thyroid nodules causing symptomatic hyperthyroidism. In children with solitary, toxic unilobar adenomas, Lobectomy or isthumusectomy (if the nodule is in the isthumus), is the treatment of choice. Just like in Graves, the patients must be rendered euthyroid both clinically and biochemically before surgery to avoid thyroid storm. Recurrent laryngeal nerve injury and bleeding are the risks involved with lobectomy.

Congenital goitre can be uninodular or multinodular. When the symptoms of compression like throat discomfort (globus sensation), difficulty in swallowing, dysphonia and difficulty in breathing especially when lying down flat, are present, surgery is recommended. In the case of uninodular goitre with compression symptoms, nodulectomy can be done. In case of multinodular goitre with compression symptoms, near total or total thyroidectomy can be done.

1.11 Thyroid Disease in Pregnancy

Women in reproductive years with thyroid disease should be treated appropriately to have a successful pregnancy. In case of hyperthyroidism, in the pre-pregnancy period, surgery may be considered and thyroid functions normalised prior to planning pregnancy. Euthyroid state is achieved with anti-thyroid drugs before surgery is performed. With this definitive surgical treatment, exposure of side effects of anti-thyroid drugs during pregnancy to both mother and foetus is avoided [17]. Following surgery, once the thyroid hormone level is stabilised with hormone replacement, then the patient is cleared for pregnancy planning. However, if hyperthyroid patient is pregnant while being treated with anti-thyroid drug methimazole, it has to be replaced with Propylthiouracil (PTU) as this is safer in the first trimester of pregnancy. In the second and third trimester of pregnancy, other anti-thyroid drugs like carbimazole are preferred. However, patient should be warned about the side effects of PTU including liver disease and congenital anomalies.

During the first few weeks of pregnancy, maternal thyroid hormone is the source of brain development for the foetus. Hence the serum TSH should be maintained as close to 2.5 uIU/mL as possible with the appropriate thyroid hormone replacement, in pregnant patients with hypothyroidism.

1.12 Post Thyroidectomy Considerations

Post-op management of thyroid surgery requires thyroid hormone replacement especially if total thyroidectomy is performed. In case of hemi-thyroidectomy, the left-over thyroid gland may be able to produce the required thyroid hormone. Calcium supplementation is necessary especially when parathyroid glands are also removed, along with vitamin D for good absorption of calcium.

In case of thyroidectomy for thyroid cancer, follow up with ultrasound of thyroid, nuclear scan, serum TSH and thyroglobulin levels on thyroid hormone suppression treatment are monitored for recurrence. Further management with repeat surgery, radioactive iodine (if scan shows uptake) chemotherapy and external radiotherapy are done as per results [18].

References

1. Unnikrishnan AG, Menon UV. Thyroid disorders in India: an epidemiological perspective. Indian J Endocr Metab. 2011;15:S78–81. https://doi.org/10.4103/2230-8210.83329.
2. Gore RW, Pandey R, Gupta DO. Incidence of thyroid disorders in Central India: retrospective analysis at rural tertiary care hospital. Galore Int J Health Sci Res. 2019;4(4):76–80.
3. Unnikrishnan AG, Kalra S, Sahay RK, Bantwal G, John M, Tewari N. Prevalence of hypothyroidism in adults: an epidemiological study in eight cities of India. Indian J Endocrinol Metab. 2013;17(4):647–52. https://doi.org/10.4103/2230-8210.113755.
4. Puneet G, Nishant R, Subhash G, Sharma AK, Sandeep G, Nishesh J, et al. Goiter prevalence and thyroid autoimmunity in school children of Delhi. Indian J Endocr Metab. 2020;24(2):202–5. https://doi.org/10.4103/ijem.IJEM_645_19.
5. Zimmermann MB, Boelaert K. Iodine deficiency and thyroid disorders. Lancet Diabetes Endocrinol. 2015;3(4):P286–95. https://doi.org/10.1016/S2213-8587(14)70225-6.
6. https://emedicine.medscape.com/article/121865-overview.
7. Pradeep PV, Agarwal A, Baxi M, Agarwal G, Gupta SK, Mishra SK. Safety and efficacy of surgical management of hyperthyroidism: 15-year experience from a tertiary care center in a developing country. World J Surg. 2007;31(2):306–12; discussion 313. https://doi.org/10.1007/s00268-006-0572-9.
8. Subasree S. Prevalence of thyroid disorders in India: an overview. Res J Pharm and Tech. 2014;7(10):1165–8.
9. Sekkath Veedu J, Wang K, Lei F, Chen Q, Huang B, Mathew A. Trends in thyroid cancer incidence in India. J Clin Oncol. 2018;36(15_suppl):e18095. https://doi.org/10.1200/JCO.2018.36.15_suppl.e18095.
10. DeGroot LJ. The non-thyroidal illness syndrome. In: Feingold KR, Anawalt B, Boyce A, et al., editors. Endotext. South Dartmouth, MA: MDText.com, Inc.; 2000. https://www.ncbi.nlm.nih.gov/books/NBK285570/.
11. Breuer C, Tuggle C, Solomon D, Sosa JA. Pediatric thyroid disease: when is surgery necessary, and who should be operating on our children? J Clin Res Pediatr Endocrinol. 2013;5(Suppl 1):79–85. https://doi.org/10.4274/jcrpe.817.
12. Agrawal P, Philip R, Saran S, Gutch M, Razi MS, Agroiya P, et al. Congenital hypothyroidism. Indian J of Endocr met. 2015;19(2):221–7.
13. Kriti J, Rishi B, Ujjal P, Preeti D. Consumptive hypothyroidism due to diffuse hepatic hemangiomas treated with propranolol therapy. Indian Pediatr. 2020;57:75–6.
14. Moutusi R, Debmalya S. Juvenile hypothyroidism: a clinical perspective from Eastern India. Indian J of Endocr Met. 2020;24(3):260–4.
15. Indumathi CK, Bantwal G, Patil M. Primary hypothyroidism with precocious puberty and bilateral cystic ovaries. Indian J Pediatr. 2007;74(8):781–3. https://doi.org/10.1007/s12098-007-0140-9.
16. Delshad H, Takyar M. Long-term Antithyroid treatment in pediatric and juvenile graves' disease. Int J Endocrinol Metab. 2020;18(Suppl):e106491. https://doi.org/10.5812/ijem.106491.
17. Francis T, Francis N, Lazarus JH, Okosieme OE. Safety of antithyroid drugs in pregnancy: update and therapy implications. Expert Opin Drug Saf. 2020;19(5):565–76. https://doi.org/10.1080/14740338.2020.1748007. Epub 2020 Apr 1.
18. Haugen BR, Alexander EK, Bible KC, Doherty GM, Mandel SJ, Nikiforov YE, et al. 2015 American Thyroid Association management guidelines for adult patients with thyroid nodules and differentiated thyroid cancer: the American Thyroid Association guidelines task force on thyroid nodules and differentiated thyroid cancer. Thyroid. 2016;26(1):1.

Solitary Thyroid Nodule

2

Loreno E. Enny, Kul Ranjan Singh, and Anand Mishra

2.1 Introduction

A thyroid nodule, defined as a 'discrete lesion in the thyroid gland that is radiologically distinct from surrounding thyroid parenchyma', is a common clinical entity. It may be clinically palpable or incidentally detected on imaging. The reported prevalence of thyroid nodules on palpation is approximately 4–7% depending on age and sex and up to 19–68% on imaging [1, 2]. As a clinician, assessing the functional status of the nodule and excluding thyroid cancer (7–15%) [3] are essential clinical objectives. In India, thyroid malignancies account for 1.8% of all cancers, with about 18,600 cases diagnosed every year [4]. Women have a threefold increased incidence (10.2 per 100,000 women) compared to men. In all cases of thyroid nodules, one needs to have answers to three questions:

1. Is this nodule or swelling symptomatic or asymptomatic and noticed insidiously? Was it present for a long duration?
2. Is this secreting excess thyroid hormone?
3. Is this swelling harbouring malignancy or at risk of developing malignancy in the future?

Thyroid nodules can be symptomatic due to pressure effects or hormonal imbalance. Most thyroid nodules in the iodine-deficient regions are benign and have a 5% risk of malignancy. The following assessments are generally recommended to answer these questions:

L. E. Enny · K. R. Singh · A. Mishra (✉)
Department of Endocrine Surgery, King George's Medical University, Lucknow, Uttar Pradesh, India

C. G. Nair, S. J. Abraham (eds.), *Surgical Management of Thyroid and Parathyroid Diseases*, https://doi.org/10.1007/978-981-97-3774-1_2

1. Clinical risk assessment includes detailed history and examination.
2. Serological or hormonal assessment for thyroid hormone status.
3. Radiological risk assessment includes high-resolution ultrasound.
4. Cytological risk assessment for the nature of the nodule.
5. Molecular risk assessment in indeterminate nodules on radiology or cytology.

Most patients with thyroid nodules are asymptomatic at presentation. A decision to operate mainly depends on the presence of compressive symptoms, concern for malignancy and the patient's choice.

2.2 Clinical Evaluation

A detailed history, good physical examination, proper imaging and fine needle aspiration biopsies (FNAB) are essential in evaluating patients with thyroid nodules. Differentiating medical and surgical diseases is the first step in evaluation. A majority of Indian patients have a sizeable palpable thyroid nodule or have symptoms due to pressure effects at presentation. A small proportion of patients report to the hospital with an incidental nodule detected on imaging for other reasons.

2.3 History

At initial presentation a detailed and relevant history, including age, gender, onset of the swelling in the neck, its duration, association with pain (acute onset pain which may indicate bleeding or acute thyroiditis), severe pain with dysphagia and hoarseness (infiltration of nerves from thyroid cancers), any recent change in size or rapid growth of nodule (haemorrhage or malignancy, presence of lymph node swelling, compressive symptoms including dry non-productive cough, strider and dyspnoea needs to be obtained.

A detailed history of symptoms of hormonal imbalance needs to be elicited. Fatigue, sensitivity to cold, weight gain and constipation indicate hypothyroidism, but weight loss, palpitation, irritability, increased appetite, and occasional diarrhoea are suggestive of hyperthyroidism. However, a marginal variation in hormone production remains asymptomatic, and that is common with hypothyroidism. A detailed history of malignancy, including a history of radiation exposure and a family history of thyroid nodules, needs to be included.

Benign thyroid diseases are frequently observed in families, but the exact hereditary root is uncertain. This could be more likely because they share similar lifestyles and food. Medullary thyroid cancer can be isolated and sporadic, but there is an increasing detection of inheritance through germline active RET protooncogene mutations. Rarely non-medullary thyroid cancers can be part of hereditary cancer syndromes like Cowden syndrome.

2.4 Physical Examination

A proper and detailed head and neck examination through inspection and palpation is of utmost importance at initial presentation, focusing mainly on the thyroid gland and the draining lymph nodes in the cervical region. The location, size, shape, surface, borders, consistency, number, tenderness of the nodule and presence of cervical lymph nodes are noted. Findings that may suggest hyperthyroidism or hypothyroidism on physical examination also need to be elicited.

A relevant physical examination that may point towards malignancy includes

1. Nodule size of ≥4 cm (19.3% risk of malignancy [5])
2. Hard to palpation
3. Fixity to surrounding structures
4. Presence of cervical lymph nodes
5. Recurrent laryngeal nerve involvement

The presence of cervical lymphadenopathy and vocal cord immobility in patients with thyroid nodules has a 100% positive predictive value for thyroid malignancy [6].

Risk Factors: There is a threefold increased prevalence of thyroid nodules in females, especially during pregnancy and in multiparous women, and may be attributed to the effects of oestrogen and progesterone [7]. The prevalence of thyroid nodules increases with age. A high goitre rate is also reported more commonly in an iodine-deficient area and in people who consume certain goitrogenic foods, including cabbage, millet, broccoli, etc. Cigarette smoking inhibits iodine uptake and organification due to thiocyanate derived from cyanide in cigarettes and is a predisposing factor for the development of goitre [8]. Obesity is also associated with an increased risk of thyroid nodules and cancer. Obese patients have advanced-stage and aggressive thyroid cancer features. A systemic review of 21 studies by Schmid et al. in 2015 showed a 25% and 55% increased risk for thyroid cancer in overweight and obese patients, respectively [9]. Tobacco and alcohol use have been shown to have an inverse relation with thyroid goitre [10].

Thyroid autoimmunity is frequently associated with thyroid nodules. In 10–31% of patients with thyroid nodules, there is associated Grave's disease. In some studies, the prevalence of thyroid autoimmunity is found to be higher in papillary thyroid cancer than in benign thyroid nodules. A meta-analysis of 10,648 cases of PTC showed that Hashimoto's thyroiditis was more prevalent in PTCs than in benign thyroid nodules [11].

Exposure to ionising radiation has been commonly demonstrated with an increased risk of thyroid cancer, especially when the direction was to a larger dose at an earlier age. This risk of developing thyroid cancer reaches a peak 15–19 years after the exposure. In a systemic review and meta-analysis, the overall exposure to diagnostic radiation was associated with a significantly increased risk of thyroid cancer [12].

A family history of thyroid cancer has been associated with a tenfold increased risk of non-medullary thyroid cancer. The familial risk for papillary carcinoma was 3.21 and 6.24, respectively, in a population-based study when a parent and a sibling were diagnosed with thyroid cancers [13]. Familial differentiated thyroid cancer may also arise as part of cancer syndrome, including Werner syndrome, Cowden's, FAP syndrome, and Carney complex. A substantial risk factor for malignancy is a personal or family history of MEN2 or FMTC.

Clinical Diagnosis: Diagnosis of a thyroid nodule is based on three criteria, namely anatomical features, hormonal profile and cytological features. The clinical examination helps to underscore the probability of a solitary nodule, multinodularity or diffuse enlargement apart from fixity to neighbouring structures and enlarged lymph nodes. Routinely performed estimation of thyrotropin (TSH) and Free Thyroxine (FT4) categorises the hormonal status to overt hyperthyroidism, subclinical hyperthyroidism, overt hypothyroidism, subclinical hypothyroidism and euthyroid state.

The nature of the pathology of thyroid nodules can broadly be classified into three types: benign, suspicious of malignancy, or malignant. Combining the above three parameters leads to diagnosis (Figs. 2.1 and 2.2). Suffixes like cervical lymph node palpable and retrosternal extension can be added. The further evaluation of hormonal profile, radiological features or fine needle aspiration cytology is based on this concept, which is why it is called a triple assessment.

Fig. 2.1 Diagnosis (CAP) of thyroid nodule

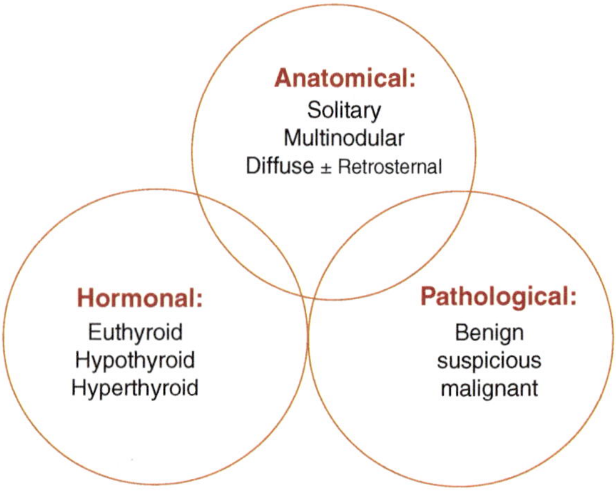

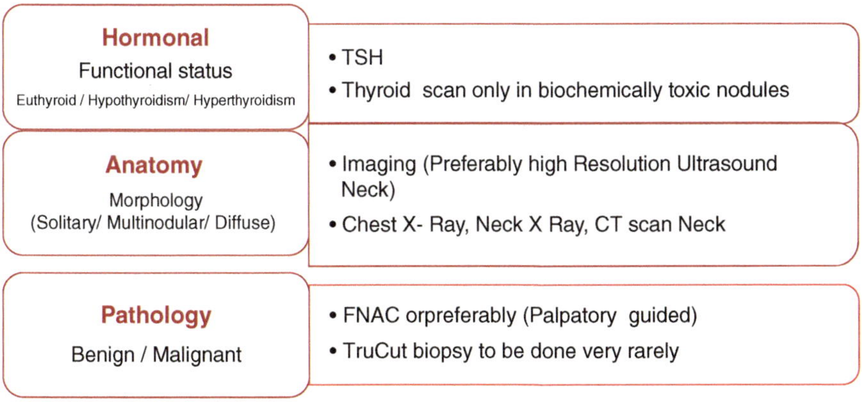

Fig. 2.2 Diagnostic work up of thyroid nodule

2.5 Serum Thyrotropin and Thyroid Hormones

The first laboratory investigation that should be obtained in a patient with thyroid nodule during initial evaluation is serum thyrotropin as its value will indicate whether the nodule is hyperfunctioning, which is seen in 10% of all nodules [14], hypo functioning or iso-functioning. When serum thyrotropin is subnormal, a free thyrotropin and total or free triiodothyronine should be measured apart from a radionuclide scan to document the functional status of the nodule. When the serum thyrotropin value is higher than the normal reference range, anti-thyroid peroxidase (anti-TPO) antibodies may be measured to evaluate for the presence of autoimmune (Hashimoto) thyroiditis [15].

2.6 Serum Thyroglobulin

Measurement of thyroglobulin in postoperative monitoring of residual, recurrent or metastatic disease in differentiated thyroid cancer may be helpful. But values may also be elevated even in many benign thyroid disorders (e.g. multinodular goitre, thyroiditis). A routine measurement of thyroglobulin at initial thyroid nodule evaluation is not recommended.

2.7 Serum Calcitonin

Calcitonin is produced by parafollicular C cells of the thyroid and is a marker for medullary thyroid carcinoma (MTC). Although routine evaluation of calcitonin may detect early MTC or C-cell hyperplasia at an early stage, there is no sufficient evidence to support that early detection reduces MTC-specific mortality. Recent guidelines do not recommend routine measurement of calcitonin [3]. Calcitonin measurement should be considered in the subgroup of patients whose elevated value may change the diagnostic or surgical approach. These include patients with a family history of MTC or MEN 2 syndrome and patients with suspicious cytology not consistent with papillary thyroid carcinoma (PTC). If measured, an unstimulated calcitonin level of >100 pg/mL suggests medullary thyroid cancer (sensitivity of 60% and specificity of 100%) [16].

2.8 Radiological Evaluation

2.8.1 Thyroid Ultrasonography

High-resolution ultrasonography (US) is the imaging modality for thyroid nodules. Diagnostic neck ultrasound should be performed in all patients presenting with palpable thyroid nodules or thyroid nodules that are incidentally diagnosed on another imaging study like computed tomography (CT), magnetic resonance imaging (MRI), or PET CT. It is the primary tool for the initial stratification of cancer risk in thyroid nodules and guides FNA decision-making. US report should include a description of thyroid parenchyma (homogenous or heterogenous), size of the gland, size, location and sonographic features of the nodule including composition (cystic, solid or spongiform), echogenicity, margin, presence of calcifications, vascularity and shape and helps in assessing cervical lymph nodes. The sonographic features suggesting malignancy include hypoechogenicity, solid composition, taller than wider orientation, and the presence of microcalcification/broken rim calcification infiltrative or irregular margin [17, 18]. A combination of criteria in the US are used to predict the risk of malignancy in thyroid nodules, and no single measure is entirely accurate in diagnosing or predicting malignancy [18].

A Thyroid Imaging Reporting and Data System (TIRADS) has been developed on the lines of BIRADS in the breasts to predict malignancy in a thyroid nodules. Many distinct TIRAD guidelines have been described to classify thyroid nodules as benign or malignant and to recommend for or against fine needle aspiration biopsy (FNAB) of the thyroid nodule (Table 2.1) [16–19]. The American Thyroid Association (ATA) has classified the nodule into high suspicious, intermediate suspicious, low suspicious, shallow suspicious and benign categories based on US features (Table 2.2).

The American College of Radiology (ACR) recommends a point system based on five US features for systematic assessment for imaging a thyroid nodule. The sum of all the points determines the Thyroid Imaging Reporting and Data System (ACR-TIRADS) classification of thyroid nodules, their estimated risk of thyroid cancer and recommendations for FNAC or surveillance [17]. The total number of points is then used to classify nodules into TR1 (benign), TR2 (not suspicious), TR3 (mildly suspicious), TR4 (moderately suspicious), TR5 (highly suspicious) categories with probability of malignancy of 0, 3.4, 14, and 87% in categories 2, 3, 4 and 5 respectively (Tables 2.2 and 2.3).

Table 2.1 TIRADS categories based on ACR-TIRADS, K-TIRADS AND EU-TIRADS with their expected prevalence of malignancy (POM) and thyroid FNAB threshold [16, 17, 19]

System	USG pattern based on	TIRADS	Categories	POM %	FNAB threshold
ACR-TIRADS	Composition, echogenicity, shape, margin, echogenic foci	1	Benign	<2%	No biopsy
		2	Not suspicious	<2%	No biopsy
		3	Mildly suspicious	5%	≥2.5 cm
		4	Moderately suspicious	5–20%	≥1.5 cm
		5	Highly suspicious	>20%	≥1 cm
K-TIRADS	Composition, echogenicity, presence of suspicious features	1	No nodule	–	No biopsy
		2	Benign	<3%	≥ 2 cm
		3	Low suspicious	3–15%	≥1.5 cm
		4	Intermediate suspicious	15–50%	≥1 cm
		5	High suspicious	>60%	≥1 cm (>0.5 cm, selective)
EU-TIRADS	Composition, echogenicity, and risk factors	1	Normal	0	–
		2	Benign	0	No FNA
		3	Low risk	2–4%	>2 cm
		4	Intermediate risk	6–17%	>1.5 cm
		5	High risk	26–87%	>1 cm

K-TIRADS Korean Society of Thyroid Radiology Thyroid Imaging Reporting and Data System; *ACR-TIRADS* American College of Radiology TIRADS; *EU TIRADS* European Union TIRADS

Table 2.2 Risk classification of thyroid nodules based on ultrasound patterns as described by American Thyroid Association

Risk categories	High	Intermediate	Low	Very low
Characteristics	Solid, hypoechoic or partially cystic nodule with irregular margin (infiltrative, micro lobulated) or taller than wider shape or micro-calcifications or broken rim calcification or extra-thyroidal extension	Hypoechoic solid nodule	Isoechoic or hyperechoic solid nodule, or partially cystic nodule with eccentric solid areas	Spongiform or partially cystic nodules
Risk of harbouring malignancy	Up to 90%	Between 10 and 20%	Between 5 and 10%	Less than 3%

Table 2.3 The ACR-TIRADS scoring system of reporting for thyroid nodules

US features		Points
Composition	Cystic or almost completely cystic	0
	Spongiform	0
	Mixed cystic and solid	1
	Solid or almost completely solid	2
Echogenicity	Anechoic	0
	Hyper or isoechoic	1
	Hypoechoic	2
	Very hypoechoic	3
Shape	Wider than tall	0
	Taller than wide	3
Margin	Smooth	0
	Ill-defined	0
	Lobulated or irregular	2
	Extrathyroidal extension	3
Echogenic foci	None or large comet tail artefact	0
	Macrocalcification	1
	Peripheral rim calcification	2
	Punctate echogenic foci	3

2.8.2 Radioisotope Imaging

Radioisotope scanning has been used to assess the functional status of the nodule into:

1. Hyperfunctioning nodule ('hot', i.e. tracer uptake more significant than the surrounding tissue);
2. Hypo functioning nodule ('cold', i.e. tracer uptake less than the surrounding tissue); and
3. Iso functioning ('warm', uptake equal to surrounding thyroid tissue).

However, it does not determine the size of the thyroid nodule. The isotopes used for imaging are technetium (99mTc), (123I), and (121I). Hot nodules account for 5%, with the likelihood of malignancy <1%. About 80–85% of thyroid nodules are cold, and about 10% may harbour malignancy [20].

2.9 CT and MRI

Generally, CT and MRI are not part of evaluating thyroid nodules and are only helpful in particular situations. These imaging are functional when thyroid cancer is suspected to invade neighbouring structures or encase the carotid artery or is found to have bulky lymph node metastases. When a primary mediastinal goitre or mediastinal extension is suspected, CT is useful in assessing the extent of the lesion and compression of the trachea. Contrast-enhanced CT should be employed cautiously in malignancy since iodine loading will induce stunning and delay the radioiodine treatment when indicated. Radioiodine ablation is usually delayed for 1–2 months when contrast-enhanced CT is done preoperatively.

2.10 18F-Fluorodeoxyglucose Positron Emission Computed Tomography (18F-FDG-PET/CT)

Although imaging with 18F-FDG PET/CT is not currently recommended during the initial workup of thyroid nodules, there is growing evidence that PET imaging is an important tool, and its use may influence the clinical management of differentiated thyroid disease. Its use has been widely accepted in detecting recurrent DTC. The emerging role of 18F-FDG PET/CT in thyroid nodules is attributed to the clinical experience of incidentally detected FDG focal thyroid uptake on PET/CT performed for unrelated non-thyroidal purposes [21]. Use of 18F-FDG PET/CT has also been shown to increase the diagnostic accuracy, especially in patients with thyroid nodule with indeterminate cytology. Vriens and colleagues have reported the pooled sensitivity, specificity, NPV, and positive predictive value of FDG-PET were 95%, 48%, 96% and 39%, respectively. A positive FDG-PET scan increases the possibility of malignancy in these patients from 25.8 to 38.7% [22].

2.11 Cytological Evaluation

Aspiration cytology has emerged as the most critical decision-making tool in managing thyroid nodules.

FNAC biopsies provide the most valuable, cost-effective and definitive diagnostic information for evaluating thyroid nodules. It is considered the most reliable technique in differentiating malignant from benign thyroid nodules. Studies have shown that even in the experienced hands, the rate of non-contributory reports may reach up to 10% [23]. The reported crude sensitivity and specificity were 65–98% and 72–100%, respectively [24]. Smaller lesions (<10 mm) and larger lesions (>30 mm) may have 1–5% negative reports [25]. but a targeted aspiration reduces the issue to some extent. Another hindrance is the more significant cystic components (25–50%) and the nodules placed in the posterior aspects of the lobes [26].

Previously, the cytology reports were confusing and were not reasonably translated to routine practical management. A standardised reporting system was introduced in 2007, popularly referred to as (Bethesda System for Reporting Thyroid Cytopathology) and was recently revised in 2016.

Over the past few years, to address the variability and standardise the reporting of thyroid cytopathology, a criteria system (Bethesda System for Reporting Thyroid Cytopathology) was introduced in 2007 and revised in 2016.

Bethesda system of reporting broadly categorises the nodules into six categories and an estimated risk of malignancy in each type is now known [27–29] (Table 2.4). The newer recommendations elaborate on the possible management

Table 2.4 Risk of malignancy in first and second editions of the Bethesda System for Reporting Thyroid Cytopathology

Bethesda classification	Diagnostic category	Risk of malignancy, first edition %	Risk of malignancy, second edition %
1	Nondiagnostic or unsatisfactory • Cyst fluid only • Obscuring blood • Insufficient number of follicular cells	1–4	5–10
2	Benign • Follicular nodule (adenomatoid and colloid nodule) • Chronic lymphocytic thyroiditis • Granulomatous thyroiditis	0–3	0–3
3	AUS/FLUS • Focal nuclear atypia • Microfollicular pattern in a hypocellular specimen • Predominance of Hurthle cells	5–15	10–30
4	FN/SFN • Crowded and overlapping follicular cells some or most of which are arranged as micro follicles	15–30	25–40
5	Suspicious for malignancy • Subtle and focal nuclear and architectural changes of malignancy	60–75	50–75
6	Malignant	97–99	97–99

protocol for the indeterminate category of cytology. The updated classification of thyroid cancers has recognised a new variety of non-invasive follicular thyroid neoplasms with papillary-like nuclear features (NIFTP), which is thought to represent an early stage of invasive encapsulated follicular variant of papillary cancer with shallow malignant potential [3]. Besides this system, there are UK and Italian categorisations of FNAC reporting, but they are not as popular as the Bethesda system (Table 2.5). In the case of patients with multi-nodular goitre, aspiration is generally done from nodules >10 mm in size with suspicious features on ultrasound imaging or from a cold nodule on scintigraphy.

Table 2.5 Comparison of the Italian AME Consensus, UK-RC Path and Bethesda systems for classification and reporting of thyroid fine needle aspiration cytology results

Italian Consensus, 2014	UK-RC path	Bethesda system
TIR 1. Non-diagnostic TIR 1c. Non-diagnostic cystic	Thy 1. Non-diagnostic Thy 1c. Unsatisfactory, consistent with cyst	I: Non-diagnostic or cystic
TIR 2. Non-malignant	Thy 2. Non-neoplastic	II: Benign
TIR 3A. Low-risk indeterminate lesion TIR 3B. High-risk indeterminate lesion	Thy 3a. Neoplasm possible: atypia Thy 3f. Neoplasm possible: suggestive of follicular neoplasm	III: AUS/FLUS atypia or follicular lesion of undetermined significance
TIR 4. Suspicious for malignancy	Thy 4. Suspicious for malignancy	IV. Follicular neoplasm or suspicious for follicular neoplasm
TIR 5. Malignant	Thy 5. Malignant	V. Suspicious for malignancy
–	–	VI. Malignant

2.12 Molecular Assessment

There is still a grey area in managing thyroid nodules with Bethesda III and IV cytological features, otherwise called the indeterminate category. The routine practice is to do a repeat aspiration under guidance. If cytological study remains non-contributory and ultrasound features are suspicious, a diagnostic lobectomy was resorted to.

After the genetic changes in differentiated thyroid cancers were established, molecular testing was incorporated into aspiration studies, which improved diagnostic accuracy. The new studies are broadly known as rule-in studies, indicating the possibility of cancer, and rule-out studies, which may exclude chances of cancer. The rule in tests include mutation analysis of set genes in the aspirated cells, a seven-gene panel (BRAF, H-RAS, N-RAS, K-RAS, RET/PTC1, RET/PTC3, PAX8/PPARγ) along with P53 and TERT gene. The presence of a mutation in BRAF, TERT, and P53 is consistently associated with thyroid cancer. The seven gene panel was found to have 95% specificity but a poor sensitivity (48%).

The two most common molecular tests are mutation analysis and gene expression analysis. Mutation analysis or testing also termed a rule in test analysis mutation in several genes, including the seven gene panel (BRAF, H-RAS, N-RAS, K-RAS, RET/PTC1, RET/PTC3, PAX8/PPARγ) along with P53 and TERT gene. The presence of a mutation in BRAF, TERT, and P53 is consistently associated with thyroid cancer. In a large prospective study on 513 nodules with Bethesda III, IV, and V cytology, the sensitivity and specificity were 63% and 99%, respectively [30]. There are many commercially available comprehensive packages for molecular study.

1. The Afirma gene expression classifier (GEC) is a rule-out test panel and examines 167 genes associated with thyroid cancer [31]. The test panel was recently updated from a microarray mRNA platform to next-generation RNA

sequencing, which utilises (NGS) platform. Thyroid nodules with Bethesda III and IV cytological features shall be observed if the GEC panel shows benign results.
2. The Thyroid Sequencing test (ThyroSeq) is a rule-in test protocol based on detecting cancer-associated molecular alterations in cell D3NA and RNA. The version included a 7-gene panel (mutations-BRAF, N-/H-/K-RAS, translocations RET/PTC and PAX8/PPAR), but the 2013 version included a 13-gene panel. ThyroSeq v2, 2014 version has a 56-gene panel analysing additional point mutations and gene fusions. The 2017 version of ThyroSeq v3 includes more than 12,000 mutation hotspots and 120 gene fusion types. Now, this panel has an improved sensitivity and specificity in detecting all types of thyroid cancers. In a prospective blinded multicentre study by Steward et al., ThyroSeq v3 demonstrated a sensitivity of 91%, specificity of 85%, PPV of 64% and NPV of 97% in Bethesda III nodules and sensitivity of 97%, specificity of 75%, PPV of 68% and NPV 98% in Bethesda IV nodules [31].
3. ThyGenX is a targeted NGS test that assays for mutations in five genes (BRAF, KRAS, HRAS, NRAS, and PIK3CA) and three gene fusions (RET-PTC1, RET-PTC3, and PAX8-PPARG) associated with thyroid cancers.
4. ThyraMIR measures the expression levels of ten microRNAs (miRNAs) and gives a risk-based classification of the nodule based on the miRNA profile.

2.13 Decision-Making and Management

Management of the patients with thyroid nodules depends on various factors, including size of the nodule, symptomatology, ultrasound and FNAC findings and patient's choice. Generally, surgery is recommended in patients with compressive symptoms, hyper-functioning nodules and nodules with suspicious or proven malignancy. For patients with unilateral compressive nodule and of benign cytology, hemithyroidectomy is preferred and for those with bilateral compressive goitre, total-thyroidectomy is recommended.

For a non-diagnostic nodule based on Bethesda classification, repeat ultrasound-guided FNAC is advised and preferably within 3–6 months to avoid a false positive result, and if it again comes out non-diagnostic, patients can be either kept on close follow-up with clinical assessment and ultrasound periodically or should be considered for thyroid lobectomy based on patient's preference and if the nodule shows high suspicious features on ultrasound (Figs. 2.3 and 2.4).

For those patients kept on follow-up, thyroid lobectomy is recommended if the nodule growth is >20% in two dimensions and >50% increase in volume. Patients with benign cytology should be kept on close follow-up with periodic

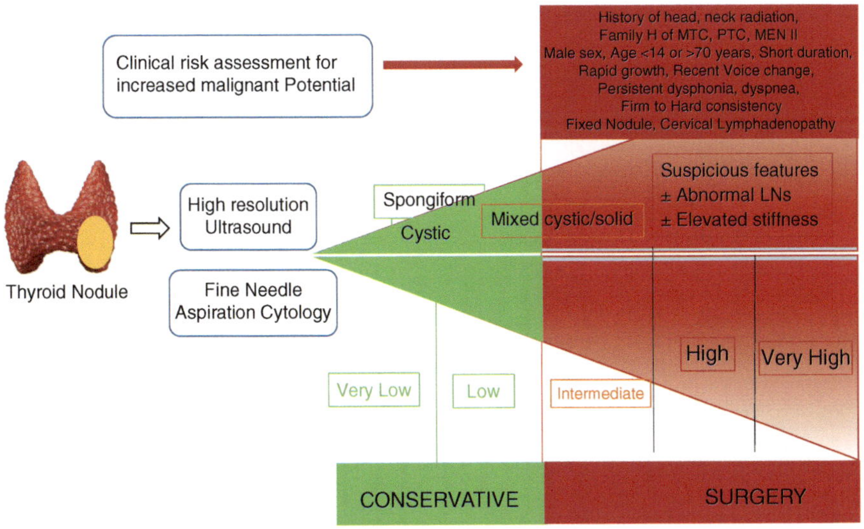

Fig. 2.3 Algorithm of work up and management of thyroid nodule

clinical and ultrasound evaluations. The interval for repeat USG may be adjusted based on the USG risk group. For those with high sonographic suspicion, repeat ultrasound should be done within 3–6 months and repeat FNAB within 12 months. For nodules with low or intermediate suspicion for malignancy, repeat USG should be repeated within 12–24 months. For nodules with very low suspicion, frequent repeat USG is not usually needed but may be repeated after 2 years or whenever a patient is symptomatic or if there is an increase in the size of the nodule. On repeat ultrasound, if the nodule shows >50% change in volume or >20% increase in two dimensions, repeat FNA, preferably USG guided, is advised [3].

These guidelines and recommendations must also take into account the patient's preference. In a remote area where the follow-up is not so robust and if the patient desire surgery due to fear of malignancy, thyroid lobectomy or total thyroidectomy can be offered depending on the clinical risk factors, sonographic features, number and site of involvement.

If the cytology is suspicious or malignancy (Bethesda 5 and 6), the preferred or recommended management is hemi or total thyroidectomy ± lymph node dissection depending on the clinical risk factor, sonographic features and molecular testing. Small intrathyroidal nodules of <1 cm could undergo active surveillance (Figs. 2.5 and 2.6) [32].

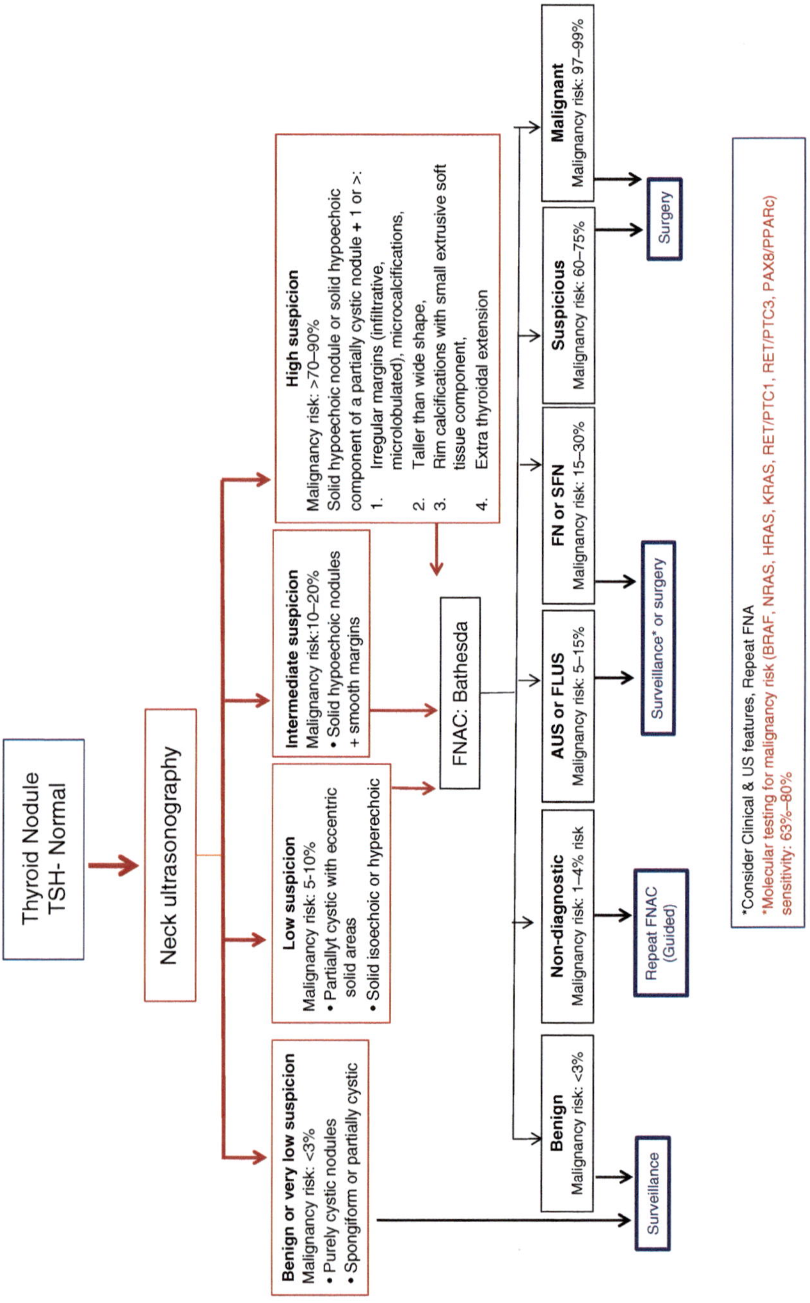

Fig. 2.4 Algorism of work up and management as per American thyroid association guidelines

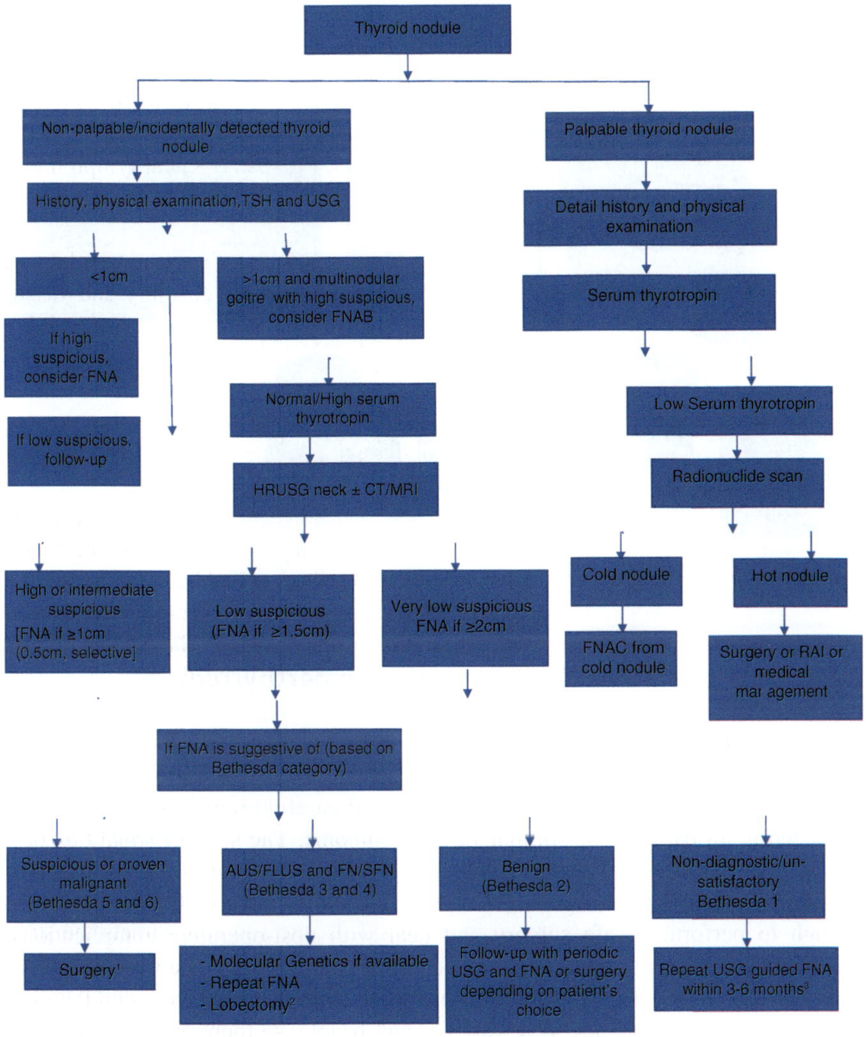

1. Extent of surgery depending on clinical risk factors, sonographic features
2. Surgery can be total thyroidectomy if Both lobes are involved and also depending on clinical risk factors
3. If repeat FNA is non-diagnostic, consider surgery or follow-up based on patient preference and risk factor

Fig. 2.5 Algorithm for thyroid nodule work up

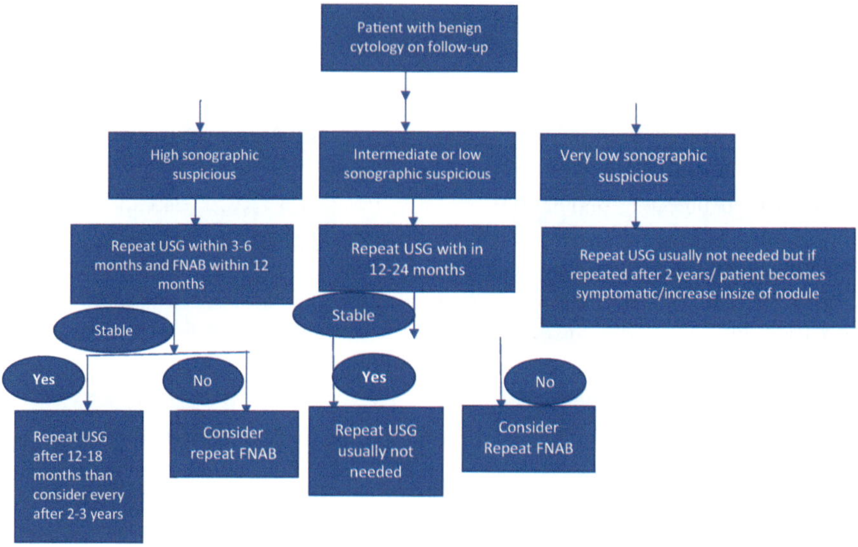

Fig. 2.6 Algorithm for patient on follow-up with benign cytology on FNAB

2.14 Pre-operative Management of Hyperthyroidism

2.14.1 Preparation

When surgery in hyperthyroid patients is planned careful preoperative preparation is needed in all patients for optimal surgical outcome. The surgery should be performed with an expert and high-volume surgeon. In literature, there are different views on high volume surgeons; however, the surgeon should be experienced enough to perform a safe surgery and deal with post-operative complications. Thyroidectomy for hyperthyroidism differs from routine since adequate preoperative control is necessary to avoid intra-operative and postoperative complications. The hyperthyroid glands are very vascular and friable, so there are more haemorrhages observed intra-operatively. The Graves' disease (GD) thyroid gland is very soft and crisp with very high risk of surface oozing during intraoperative handling. The postoperative toxic crisis is a dreaded complication, and proper preparation greatly reduces the chance of this complication.

The '**ABCD**' approach:

1. **Adequate** euthyroidsm ('**A**'): Pre-treatment with anti-thyroid drugs (ATDs) (methimazole, carbimazole, propylthiouracil) and beta-blockers (propranolol) is mandatory to achieve euthyroidism. There are different indications for drugs, and adequate doses should be used. Beta-blockers should be used in addition, as they control the peripheral effects of excess thyroid hormones, and block T4 to T3 conversion. All patients should be assessed clinically for thyroid status. They

should be asymptomatic, and pulse rate should be less than 90 beats/min. Biochemically, the thyroid function test should be normal (T4 and TSH). If TSH is low, then Free T4 should be assessed, and if it is normal, then the patient should be considered as euthyroid. It is known that TSH takes a longer time to recover.

2. To decrease intra-operative **Bleeding** (‘**B**’): Graves’ disease gland is very vascular, soft and friable, and intraoperatively, there is a risk of haemorrhage and surface oozing. Inorganic iodide decreases thyroid gland vascularity and thyroid hormone release during surgery. A saturated solution of potassium iodide (SSKI) or potassium iodine (Lugol’s solution) is available and used preoperatively for 7–10 days. It should be used for short periods as Iodide has an escape phenomenon effect (Wolff-Chaikoff effect). KI can be given as 5–7 drops (0.25–0.35 mL) of Lugol’s solution, which contains 8 mg iodide per drop, or 1–2 drops (0.05–0.1 mL) of SSKI, which contains 50 mg iodide per drop three times daily mixed in water or juice started 10 days prior to surgery.
3. **Calcium** supplementation (‘**C**’): In all patients, calcium should be supplemented adequately as these patients have some component of thyrotoxic bone disease in which bone mineral density has become low. If the patient is vitamin D deficient, it should be corrected. These measures are required to decrease the chances of post-thyroidectomy hypocalcaemia.
4. Other **Drugs** (‘**D**’): Some patients are intolerant or allergic to ATDs. Also, there may be a need for urgent thyroidectomy in some patients because of various reasons. In all these patients and in situations where rapid preparation is needed, a combination of beta-adrenergic blockade, KI, and glucocorticoids can be used. Cholestyramine can be useful in the immediate preoperative period. Glucocorticoids (Hydrocortisone 300 mg IV followed by 100 mg 8 h or dexamethasone 2 mg twice a day intravenous or oral) reduce peripheral T4 to T3 conversion and abolish the risk of adrenal insufficiency. Cholestyramine is anionic exchange resin which binds to iodothyronines in the gastrointestinal tract, decreasing serum thyroid hormone levels.

   Up to 12 g of cholestyramine can be used in divided three times doses along with thionamides and a β-adrenergic blocker. It should be reserved for severe or resistant to conventional therapy GD. Rapid preoperative preparation can be achieved by adding Ipanoic acid 500 mg twice a day and dexamethasone 1 mg BD to ATD and beta blockers. Guanethidine (30–40 mg orally 6 h) and Reserpine (2.5–5 mg IM 4 h) are useful when beta blockers are contra indicated. They decrease the availability of catecholamine.

Erbil et al. have done prospective clinical trial to see the effect of Lugol solution and concluded that preoperative Lugol solution treatment decreased rate of blood flow, thyroid vascularity, and intraoperative blood loss during thyroidectomy. However, this study had small patient number (17 patient in Lugol group, 19 in without group). The blood flow was assessed by colour flow doppler ultrasonography and microvessel density (MVD) was assessed by immunohistochemical and Western blot analysis. [33] Yilmaz et al. also performed a controlled, randomised, prospective study on 40 patients and concluded that preoperative Lugol use decreased rate of blood flow and intraoperative blood loss during surgery [34]. Nair et al. have used also in their patients iodine and lithium carbonate [35]. Hope et al. reviewed an extensive literature search on pre-operative preparation in hyperthyroid patients and reported that the evidence was very weak in literature in this field [36]. Yamanouchi et al. reviewed their patients for predicting factors for intra-operative excessive bleeding and found goitre more than 200 g was the only predictive factor for excessive bleeding and suggested that in all these patients blood transfusion should be considered [37].

2.15 Indications for Operation

The main indications for surgery in benign nodular goitre can be remembered by **5 C**s

1. **C**osmesis: Large goitres
2. **C**ontrol: Failure of medical treatment to control toxicity or as definitive treatment of toxic goitres.
3. **C**ompression: Compression of airway and superior vena cava
4. **C**ancer: Fear of cancer and occult carcinoma, malignancy proven on FNAC possible malignancy (atypical, suspicious findings on FNAC)
5. **C**ome back: Recurrence of goitre

Indications of thyroidectomy in GD patients can be remembered by **6 Cs** and include:

1. Anti-thyroid drugs **C**annot be given: Difficulty with adequate hormonal control on medications, or Intolerance, or recurrence after ATD treatment.
2. RAI **C**ontraindication: Pregnant and nursing women, large goitre with or without compressive symptoms (dysphagia, dysphonia, dyspnoea), relatively low uptake of RAI, associated thyroid nodule with confirmed or suspected thyroid malignancy.
3. Patients with moderate-to-severe active Graves' orbitopathy **C**oexisting.
4. Associated **C**oexisting disease like periodic paralysis.
5. Other **C**onditions: Young or paediatric patients, if a woman is planning a pregnancy in the next 6 months, refusal of RAI or patient from locality with lack of facilities for RAI, patient prefers surgery over medical management.
6. **C**igarette smokers: Increased risk of exacerbation of eye disease after definitive treatment with radioactive iodine.

2.16 Therapy with Radioiodine

The indications of thyroidectomy are very well defined however in situations of associated multiple morbidities it becomes very risky. Radioiodine therapy (RIT) or radioactive iodine (RAI) therapy is an option only in patients with high risk for anaesthesia. RIT may reduce the size of goitre up to 60% but there is risk of developing temporary mild thyrotoxicosis in first 2 weeks of treatment. To prevent this, RIT should be used under cover of glucocorticoid and beta blockers. Patients can have acute adverse effects like painful transient thyroiditis, feeling of compression of trachea and symptoms related to the cardiovascular system. In long term patient develop unpredictable hypothyroidism (up to 45%). There is always a little risk of 1.6% of cancer development in body [38, 39]. Simultaneous use of recombinant TSH (rhTSH) increase accumulation of RAI two to four times [40]. One to two injection of rhTSH (0.1–0.3 mg) should be administered 24 h prior to RIT.

In summary, RIT results in:

1. RAI can cause volume reduction of 33–66% in 80% of patients
2. It improves dysphagia or dyspnoea in 70–90% of patients
3. Post RAI hypothyroidism is observed in 60% of patients at 8 years
4. Post RAI Graves' disease is seen in 10% of patients
5. Post RAI lifetime cancer risk is 1.6%

RIT is also a definitive method of choice in patients with hyperthyroidism especial so in Graves' disease. It is used also in persistent GD, toxic adenoma and toxic multi nodular goitre. The trapped iodine (I^{131}) emits radiation intra-parenchymally and cause destruction of thyrotropes and resulting in thyroid gland. RIT is indicated in persistent GD post ATDs which are small goitres (40–60 mL volume), preferably without ocular involvement. It should be given under steroid cover as already discussed (0.5 mg/kg of prednisolone for 1–3 months). RAI is contraindicated in pregnancy, lactation, suspected or proven thyroid malignancy, paediatric age group [41].

2.17 Summary

Thyroid nodule is a common clinical entity. It can be either palpable or incidentally detected on imaging done for other non-thyroidal purpose. The clinical importance of thyroid nodule is to differentiate benign from malignant thyroid nodule. TIRADs guidelines have been adapted to classify thyroid nodule and this helps in deciding on further testing for FNAB. Management of thyroid nodule is based on the different clinical risk factors, sonographic image findings, FNAB findings and patient's choice. Molecular genetics is being increasingly used to rule in or rule out malignancy and has been found to be helpful for decision making in the primary surgical treatment, especially in a nodule with indeterminate cytology.

References

1. Singer PA. Evaluation and management of the solitary thyroid nodule. Otolaryngol Clin N Am. 1996;29(4):577–91.
2. Guth S, Theune U, Aberle J, Galach A, Bamberger CM. Very high prevalence of thyroid nodules detected by high frequency (13 MHz) ultrasound examination. EurJ Clin Invest. 2009;39:699–706.

3. Haugen BR, Alexander EK, Bible KC, Doherty GM, Mandel SJ, Nikiforov YE, et al. American Thyroid Association management guidelines for adult patients with Thyroid nodules and differentiated thyroid cancer: the American Thyroid Association guidelines task force on Thyroid nodules and differentiated Thyroid cancer. Thyroid Off J Am Thyroid Assoc. 2016;26(1):1–133.
4. Bray F, Ferlay J, Soerjomataram I, Siegel RL, Torre LA, Jemal A. Global cancer statistics 2018: GLOBOCAN estimates of incidence and mortality worldwide for 36 cancers in 185 countries. CA Cancer J Clin. 2018;68(6):394–424.
5. McCoy KL, Jabbour N, Ogilvie JB, Ohori NP, Carty SE, Yim JH. The incidence of cancer and rate of false-negative cytology in thyroid nodules greater than or equal to 4 cm in size. Surgery. 2007;142(6):837–44.
6. Raza SN, Shah MD, Palme CE, Hall FT, Eski S, Freeman JL. Risk factors for well-differentiated thyroid carcinoma in patients with thyroid nodular disease. Otolaryngol Head Neck Surg. 2008;139(1):21–6.
7. Popoveniuc G, Jonklaas J, Thyroid nodules. The medical clinics of North America. Med Clin North Am. 2012;96(2):329–49.
8. Lio S, Napolitano G, Marinuzzi G, Monaco F. Role of smoking in goiter morphology and thyrotropin response to TRH in untreated goitrous women. J Endocrinol Investig. 1989;12(2):93–7.
9. Schmid D, Ricci C, Behrens G, Leitzmann MF. Adiposity and risk of thyroid cancer: a systematic review and meta-analysis. Obes Rev. 2015;16:1042–54.
10. Lee JH, Kim Y, Choi JW, Kim YS. The association between papillary thyroid carcinoma and histologically proven Hashimoto's thyroiditis: a meta-analysis. Eur J Endocrinol. 2013;168:343–9.
11. Han MA, Kim JH. Diagnostic X-ray exposure and thyroid cancer risk: systematic review and meta-analysis. Thyroid. 2018;28:220–8. https://doi.org/10.1089/thy.2017.0159.
12. Hemminki K, Eng C, Chen B. Familial risks for nonmedullary thyroid cancer. J Clin Endocrinol Metab. 2005;90:5747–53. https://doi.org/10.1210/jc.2005-0935.
13. Wong CK, Wheeler MH. Thyroid nodules: rational management. World J Surg. 2000;24(8):934–41.
14. Gharib H, Papini E, Garber JR, et al. American Association of Clinical Endocrinologists, American College of Endocrinology, and Associazione Medici Endocrinologi medical guidelines for clinical practice for the diagnosis and management of thyroid nodules—2016 update. Endocr Pract. 2016;22(5):622–39.
15. Costante G, Meringolo D, Durante C, et al. Predictive value of serum calcitonin levels for preoperative diagnosis of medullary thyroid carcinoma in a cohort of 5817 consecutive patients with thyroid nodules. J Clin Endocrinol Metab. 2007;92(2):450–5.
16. Shin JH, Baek JH, Chung J, Ha EJ, Kim J, Lee YH, et al. Ultrasonography diagnosis and imaging-based management of thyroid nodules: revised Korean Society of Thyroid Radiology consensus statement and recommendations. Korean J Radiol. 2016;17(3):370–95.
17. Tessler FN, Middleton WD, Grant EG, Hoang JK, Berland LL, Teefey SA, et al. ACR thyroid imaging, reporting and data system (TI-RADS): white paper of the ACR TI-RADS committee. J Am Coll Radiol. 2017;14(5):587–95.
18. Russ G. Risk stratification of thyroid nodules on ultrasonography with the French TI-RADS: description and reflections. Ultrasonography. 2016;35(1):25–38.
19. Russ G, Bonnema SJ, Erdogan MF, Durante C, Ngu R, Leenhardt L. European Thyroid Association guidelines for ultrasound malignancy risk stratification of thyroid nodules in adults: the EU-TIRADS. Eur Thyroid J. 2017;6(5):225–37.
20. Cases JA, Surks MI. The changing role of scintigraphy in the evaluation of thyroid nodules. Semin Nucl Med. 2000;30(2):81–7.
21. Iyer NG, Shaha AR, Silver CE, Devaney KO, Rinaldo A, Pellitteri PK, et al. Thyroid incidentalomas: to treat or not to treat. Eur Arch Otorrinolaringol. 2010;267:1019–26.
22. Vriens D, deWilt JH, van derWilt GJ, Netea-Maier RT, Oyen WJ, de Geus-Oei LF. The role of [(18) F]-2-fluoro-2-deoxy-d-glucosepositron emission tomography in thyroid nodules with indeterminate fine-needle aspiration biopsy: systematic review and metaanalysis of the literature. Cancer. 2011;117:4582–94.

23. Bojunga J, Herrmann E, Meyer G, Weber S, Zeuzem S, Friedrich-Rust M. Real-time elastography for the differentiation of benign and malignant thyroid nodules: a meta-analysis. Thyroid Off J Am Thyroid Assoc. 2010;20(10):1145–50.
24. Niedziela M. Thyroid nodules. Best Pract Res Clin Endocrinol Metab. 2014;28(2):245–77.
25. Gharib H, Goellner JR. Fine-needle aspiration biopsy of the thyroid: an appraisal. Ann Intern Med. 1993;118:282–9.
26. Tamhane S, Gharib H. Thyroid nodule update on diagnosis and management. Clin Diabetes Endocrinol. 2016;2(1):17.
27. Baloch ZW, LiVolsi VA, Asa SL, Rosai J, Merino MJ, Randolph G, Vielh P, DeMay RM, Sidawy MK, Frable WJ. Diagnostic terminology and morphologic criteria for cytologic diagnosis of thyroid lesions: a synopsis of the National Cancer Institute thyroid fine-needle aspiration state of the science conference. Diagn Cytopathol. 2008;36:425–37.
28. Crippa S, Mazzucchelli L, Cibas ES, Ali SZ. The Bethesda system for reporting thyroid fine-needle aspiration specimens. Am J Clin Pathol. 2010;134:343–4.
29. Pusztaszeri M, Rossi ED, Auger M, et al. The Bethesda system for reporting thyroid cytopathology: proposed modifications and updates for the second edition from an international panel. Acta Cytol. 2016;60:399–405.
30. Nikiforov YE, Ohori NP, Hodak SP, et al. Impact of mutational testing on the diagnosis and management of patients with cytologically indeterminate thyroid nodules: a prospective analysis of 1056 FNA samples. J Clin Endocrinol Metab. 2011;96(11):3390–7.
31. Steward DL, Carty SE, Sippel RS, et al. Performance of a multigene genomic classifier in thyroid nodules with indeterminate cytology: a prospective blinded multicenter study. JAMA Oncol. 2018;5:204.
32. Ito Y, Miyauchi A, Oda H. Low-risk papillary microcarcinoma of thyroid: a review of active surveillance. Eur J Surg Onco. 2018;44(3):307–15.
33. Erbil Y, Ozluk Y, Giriş M, Salmaslioglu A, Issever H, Barbaros U, Kapran Y, Ozarmağan S, Tezelman S. Effect of lugol solution on thyroid gland blood flow and microvessel density in the patients with graves' disease. J Clin Endocrinol Metab. 2007;92(6):2182–9. https://doi.org/10.1210/jc.2007-0229. Epub 2007 Mar 27
34. Yilmaz Y, Kamer KE, Ureyen O, Sari E, Acar T, Karahalli O. The effect of preoperative Lugol's iodine on intraoperative bleeding in patients with hyperthyroidism. Ann Med Surg (Lond). 2016;9:53–7. https://doi.org/10.1016/j.amsu.2016.06.002.
35. Nair GC, Babu MJC, Menon R, Jacob P. Preoperative preparation of hyperthyroidism for thyroidectomy—role of supersaturated iodine and lithium carbonate. Indian J Endocrinol Metab. 2018;22(3):392–6. https://doi.org/10.4103/ijem.IJEM_3_18.
36. Hope N, Kelly A. Pre-operative Lugol's iodine treatment in the management of patients undergoing thyroidectomy for graves' disease: a review of the literature. Eur Thyroid J. 2017;6(1):20–5. https://doi.org/10.1159/000450976. Epub 2016 Nov 22.
37. Yamanouchi K, Minami S, Hayashida N, Sakimura C, Kuroki T, Eguchi S. Predictive factors for intraoperative excessive bleeding in graves' disease. Asian J Surg. 2015;38(1):1–5. https://doi.org/10.1016/j.asjsur.2014.04.007. Epub 2014 Jun 14.
38. Wesche MF, Tiel-V Buul MM, Lips P, Smits NJ, Wiersinga WM. A random-ized trial comparing levothyroxine with radioactive iodine in the treatment of sporadic nontoxic goiter. J Clin Endocrinol Metab. 2001;86:998–1005.
39. Huysmans DA, Buijs WC, van de Ven MT, van den Broek WJ, Kloppenborg PW, Hermus AR, et al. Dosimetry and risk estimates of radioiodine therapy for large, multinodular goiters. J Nucl Med. 1996;37:2072–9.
40. Bonnema SJ, Fast S, Hegedüs L. The role of radioiodine therapy in benign nodular goiter. Best Pract Res Clin Endocrinol Metabol. 2014;28:619–31.
41. Ross DS, Burch HB, Cooper DS, Greenlee MC, Laurberg P, Maia AL, et al. (2016) American Thyroid Association guidelines for diagnosis and management of hyperthyroidism and other causes of thyrotoxicosis. Thyroid. 2016;26(10):1343–421.

Overview of Surgical Management of Hyperthyroidism

3

C. Gopalakrishnan Nair and Misha J. C. Babu

There is a global high prevalence of diseases of the thyroid gland, and found to be the second most common endocrine disease. An epidemiological survey in Kerala, India, showed 1.3 and 1.6% incidences of overt and subclinical hyperthyroidism, respectively [1, 2].

The first description of primary hyperthyroidism was from Caleb Hillier Parry (1755–1822) in 1786, and he gave a detailed account of exophthalmic goitre. His picturesque description of the disease is relevant even now—"eyes were protruded from their sockets, faces exhibited an appearance of agitation and distress, the heartbeat was so violent that each systole of the heart shook the whole thorax…" [3]. Robert James Graves (1796–1853) published a vivid description of exophthalmic goitre in 1833, and almost simultaneously, Adolph von Basedow (1779–1854) of Germany gave a good description of diffuse toxic goitre, and his name referred to the disease. Primary hyperthyroidism is probably unique because it has the names of three distinguished clinicians attached. However, the term hyperthyroidism was suggested by Charles Mayo in 1907. Interestingly, only two decades later, in 1924, Henry Plummer and Walter Boothby of the Mayo Clinic suggested that the thyroid liberated excessive hormones in Graves' disease.

Thyroidectomy was the chosen treatment for hyperthyroidism about half a century before medical treatment was found possible to control the disease. In 1943, Astwood reported the usefulness of thiouracil in controlling hormone synthesis, and the molecule remains a critical agent in the management of hyperthyroidism [4]. A few years later (1952), Carbimazole was introduced and is the widely used anti-thyroid drug. The use of radioiodine in hyperthyroidism was a contribution of Karl Taylor Compton

C. G. Nair (✉)
Professor of Surgery, Endocrine Surgery Division, Amrita Institute of Medical Sciences and Research Centre, Kochi, Kerala, India

M. J. C. Babu
Department of Surgery, AIMS, Kochi, Kochi, Kerala, India

C. G. Nair, S. J. Abraham (eds.), *Surgical Management of Thyroid and Parathyroid Diseases*, https://doi.org/10.1007/978-981-97-3774-1_3

from the Massachusetts Institute of Technology [5]. Hertz and Roberts of Harvard General Hospital performed the first effective radioiodine treatment in 1941 [6].

Henry Plummer's astute observation and analysis of clinical and pathological features of about 3000 operated patients paved the way to categorise hyperthyroidism. They established the existence of primary and secondary hyperthyroidism and postulated the concept of toxic nodular goitre, and Graves' diseases were distinctly different types of hyperthyroidism [7].

Based on clinical features and biochemical profile, both hyperthyroidism and hypothyroidism were classified as overt and subclinical diseases. Overt hyperthyroidism is characterised by symptoms related to common target organs, such as cardiovascular, gastrointestinal, or general metabolic disturbances and confirmed by estimation of hormonal profile. Overt hyperthyroidism is characterised by low TSH and elevated Free-thyroxine estimates (T4). The subclinical disease shows low serum TSH levels with Free Thyroxine estimates (FT4) and Tri-iodothyronine remaining normal. An accurate distinction between toxic nodular disease and Graves' disease shall be made by estimating circulating TSH receptor antibodies. Technetium 99 scintigraphy shows different uptake patterns in toxic nodular goitre and Graves' disease.

Graves' disease (GD), toxic multinodular goitre (TMNG), and toxic adenoma (TA) are three different aetiologies of hyperthyroidism acting through different pathways. GD is an autoimmune disorder where thyrotropin receptor antibodies (TR Ab) stimulate TSH receptors, causing uncontrolled hormone production. The development of thyroid nodules is a prolonged, complex process, and over time, areas of the thyroid turn autonomous and liberated from the standard regulation by thyroid stimulating hormone. Toxic adenoma is formed from genetically altered cells with somatic mutations liberated from control of TSH. Subacute thyroiditis, probably of viral origin and lymphocytic infiltration and disintegration of follicular cells releasing the stored hormones. Drugs like lithium, interferon-@, amiodaron, and tyrosine kinase inhibitors have a similar effect on the thyroid gland.

Theodor Kocher revolutionised the surgery of the thyroid gland with great precision. Surgery in thyrocardiac patients was dissuaded by even Kocher since he felt: "Excision should not be undertaken when the disease is advanced, i.e., when the pulse, besides being rapid, is also small and irregular, or when the heart is dilated and oedema is present" [8].

He advocated thyroidectomy for hyperthyroidism but recommended a staged procedure. He used to expose the thyroid gland and ligated all named arteries to diminish blood supply and removed one lobe as the second stage. He completed the procedure when necessary, with a third surgery when he removed the remaining lobe.

Charles Mayo, the father of thyroid surgery in America, initially followed Kocher's regimen of staged hemithyroidectomy procedures. But with the help of his colleague, Plummer, who initiated preoperative usage of iodine, he could reduce the mortality rate of Graves' disease considerably.

Thomas Dunhill was the first surgeon to recommend more extensive removal of thyroid tissue than hemithyroidectomy in Graves's disease, and he removed part of the other lobe also. His operation offered a chance of a better cure for Graves' disease.

Traditionally, patients with hyperthyroidism are treated with anti-thyroid drugs to make them euthyroid before surgery. The biochemical euthyroid state is ensured by estimating the serum-free T4 level and T3 level. Normalisation of serum TSH is usually delayed in Graves' disease. The first attempt to control the deleterious effects of excess circulating hormone before thyroidectomy was by Henry Plummer. He introduced the use of iodine before thyroidectomy in 1913. The widely used preparation was Lugol's solution (LS). LS was developed in 1829 by the French physician Jean Guillaume Auguste Lugol to treat tuberculosis. The solution contains 5% elemental iodine in 10% potassium iodide and distilled water, and one drop delivers 5–8 mg of iodine. More potent preparations deliver high doses of iodine and are collectively named Supersaturated Iodine preparations (SSI).

The average requirement of iodine (100–150 μg) is absorbed from dietary sources for regular synthesis of thyroxine. The iodine uptake is by an active Na/I transporter mechanism in the follicular cell membrane and is controlled by an auto-regulatory mechanism to prevent iodine overload. The autoregulation with stands excess iodine intake up to 1100 μg iodine per day. The autoregulation is disorganised in patients with Hashimoto's thyroiditis, treated GD, and in post-thyroidectomy remnants.

A sudden iodine overload in the iodine deficiency state may induce hyperthyroidism (Jod-Basedow effect), but the gland resumes a euthyroid state when the supply is withdrawn. A short-term excess of iodine suppresses hormone synthesis (Wolff-Chaikoff effect), which is mediated by several mechanisms, including suppression of the active transporter mechanism and the thyroperoxidase enzyme. Excess iodine temporarily blocks the hormone release. The follicular cells escape from acute effects, but continued suppression of sodium/iodide symporter function occasionally persists. The cells attain normality slowly, but the adaptation phenomenon may start 2 days after iodine loading, and the release is complete in 4–11 days [9]. However, a few remain suppressed for a long time. Plummer found reduced blood flow in the thyroid gland prepared with iodine. SSI induces blood flow regulation, probably due to a reduction in VEGF and interleukin-16 [10, 11].

American Thyroid Association recommends 5–7 drops of Lugol's Solution thrice daily or 1–2 drops of Super Saturated Potassium Iodide (SSKI) (50–100 mg iodide) 10 days before thyroidectomy. Five drops of LS thrice daily equals 100.5 mg of elemental iodine. Many surgeons use iodine preparations preoperatively to reduce blood loss during operation. The authors of the text do not endorse the view since preoperative control of the hyperthyroid state with antithyroid drugs seems effective in minimising operative blood loss. There is no significant difference in blood loss between nontoxic nodular and toxic goitres when toxicity is adequately controlled.

Occasional patients are refractory to thiouracils in the possible maximal doses, allergic to thiouracils, or develop side effects. A possible reason for this poor uptake of thiouracils, even at a high dose (Lie et al. [12]). The explanations are rapid drug metabolism and the presence of drug antibodies. GD patients with excess T3 in circulation are also found refractory to thioamides.

Preoperative preparation of such patients is challenging and requires close monitoring in an inpatient setup. Supersaturated iodine preparations, cholestyramine, and steroids are alternate agents in such conditions.

Cholestyramine: About 20% of circulating thyroxine is metabolised in the liver, conjugated to glucuronides or sulphate, and enters the enterohepatic circulation pathway. In hyperthyroidism, the enterohepatic circulation is enhanced [13, 14]. Cholestyramine favours faecal excretion of T4, breaks excess enterohepatic circulation and lowers serum levels. The action seems sustained and is used as an adjunct with thionamides in refractory cases. The first report on the usefulness of cholestyramine in controlling hyperthyroidism was noted in 1993 [15]. However, the effect of cholestyramine as an adjunct in preoperative preparation of refractory Graves' disease is not convincing.

The effect of dexamethasone in Graves' disease and normal thyroid was studied by Donald Williams et al. in 1975, who found that 3 mg of the drug given sixth hourly for a day significantly reduced serum levels of T4, T3, and thyroglobulin within 24 h. The effect lasted for 4–6 days, but the impact on normal thyroid is insignificant. Dexamethasone and other steroids affect the peripheral conversion of T4 to T3 but do not suppress the effect of endogenous TSH [16]. There are anecdotal reports of dexamethasone as an adjunct in the treatment of refractory hyperthyroidism.

Lithium carbonate is a widely used drug in manic-depressive diseases, and its potential impact on thyroid function is well known. Lithium carbonate was used occasionally as an alternative when thioamides induced hepatic injury. Lithium carbonate (50–75 mg daily) as a long-term alternate treatment for patients with hepatotoxicity or leukopenia was tried by Zheng et al. [17]. Lithium is absorbed in thyroid follicular cells, inhibiting iodine uptake and thyroxine synthesis. Lithium also alters thyroglobulin structure and inhibits thyroxine synthesis [18].

A short course of lithium was administered to potentiate I131 in the management of Graves' disease. Sustained release of lithium carbonate (tablets 400 mg twice daily for 5–6 days) is an adequate preoperative preparation for Graves' disease and is unlikely to induce any toxicity. A cocktail of lithium, dexamethasone, and beta-blockers was used for preoperative preparation with thionamides in refractory patients [19].

Thyroidectomy is one of the treatment options for the management of hyperthyroidism and is usually resorted to as the last option in India. Generally, medical management with anti-thyroid drugs is the first line of management. The majority of patients are treated with radioiodine when long-term medical management fails to control relapses. Thyroidectomy is generally recommended for patients with large volume goitres, suspected or confirmed coexisting cancers, relapses following radioiodine, or emergent control of toxicity.

Thyroidectomy for hyperthyroidism is safe and has the advantage of detecting incidental carcinomas. The outcome of coexisting carcinoma is debated, but we observed disease progression in a considerable number of patients.

Incidences of transient and permanent hypocalcaemia were found to be high following thyroidectomy for Graves' disease.

References

1. Unnikrishnan AG, Menon UV. Thyroid disorders in India: an epidemiological perspective. Indian J Endocrinol Metab. 2011;15(Suppl 2):S78–81. https://doi.org/10.4103/2230-8210.83329.
2. Usha Menon V, Sundaram KR, Unnikrishnan AG, Jayakumar RV, Nair V, Kumar H. High prevalence of undetected thyroid disorders in an iodine-sufficient adult south Indian population. J Indian Med Assoc. 2009;107(2):72–7.
3. Parry CH. Collections from the unpublished medical writings of the late Caleb Hillier Parry (volume 2). London: Underwoods; 1825. p. 111.
4. Astwood EB. Treatment of hyperthyroidism with thiourea and thiouracil. JAMA J Am Med Assoc. 1943;122:78–85.
5. Ahmed AM, Ahmed NH. History of disorders of thyroid dysfunction. East Mediterr Health J. 2005;11(3):459–69.
6. Sawin CT, Becker DV. Radioiodine and the treatment of hyperthyroidism: the early history. Thyroid. 1997;7:163–76.
7. Miller M. Plummer's disease. Med Clin North Am. 1975;59(5):1203–16.
8. Textbook of operative surgery. [Trans.]. 5th ed. London: Adam & Charles Black; 1911. p. 467.
9. Eng PH, Cardona GR, Fang SL, Previti M, Alex S, Carrasco N, Chin WW, Braverman LE. Escape from the acute Wolff-Chaikoff effect is associated with a decrease in thyroid sodium/iodide symporter messenger ribonucleic acid and protein. Endocrinology. 1999;140(8):3404–10.
10. Emerson CH, Anderson AJ, Howard WJ, Utiger RD. Serum thyroxine and triiodothyronine concentrations during iodide treatment of hyperthyroidism. J Clin Endocrinol Metab. 1975;40(1):33–6.
11. Calissendorff J, Falhammar H. Lugol's solution and other iodide preparations: perspectives and research directions in graves' disease. Endocrine. 2017;58(3):467–73. https://doi.org/10.1007/s12020-017-1461.
12. Li H, Okuda J, Akamizu T, Mori T. A hyperthyroid patient with graves' disease who was strongly resistant to methimazole: investigation on possible mechanisms of the resistance. Endocr J. 1995;42(5):697–704.
13. Kohrle J, Hesch RD, Leonard JL. Intracellular pathways of iodothyronine metabolism. In: Braverman LE, Utiger RD, editors. The thyroid, a clinical and fundamental text. 6th ed. Philadelphia: JB Lippincott Company; 1991. p. 144–89.
14. Hillier AP. Autoregulation of thyroxine secretion into bile. J Physiol. 1972;221(2):471–6.
15. Shakir KMM, Michaels RD, Hays JH, Potter BB. The use of bile acid sequestrants to lower serum thyroid hormones in iatrogenic hyperthyroidism. Ann Intern Med. 1993;118:112–3.
16. Williams DE, Chopra IJ, Orgiazzi J, Solomon DH. Acute effects of corticosteroids on thyroid activity in graves' disease. J Clin Endocrinol Metab. 1975;41(2):354–61. https://doi.org/10.1210/jcem-41-2-354.
17. Parker PE, Walter-Ryan WG, Pittman CS, Folks DG. Lithium treatment of hyperthyroidism and mania. J Clin Psychiatry. 1986;47(5):264–6.
18. Lazarus JH. The effects of lithium therapy on thyroid and thyrotropin-releasing hormone. Thyroid. 1998;8(10):909–13. https://doi.org/10.1089/thy.1998.8.909.
19. Nair GC, Babu MJC, Menon R, Jacob P. Preoperative preparation of hyperthyroidism for thyroidectomy—role of supersaturated iodine and lithium carbonate. Indian. J Endocrinol Metab. 2018;22(3):392–6.

Anatomy of Thyroid and Parathyroid Glands

4

C. Gopalakrishnan Nair

The thyroid gland is placed on the front of the lower neck, close to the lateral aspects of the larynx and trachea. The isthmus bridging the lobes crosses the second and third rings of the trachea. The gland is covered anteriorly by strap muscles, an investing layer of deep fascia and subcutaneous tissue. The superficial fascia of the neck is a layer of loose connective tissue extending to the face, which is embedded in the voluntary muscles of facial expression and the platysma. The subcutaneous nerves, venules, lymphatics, and portions of the anterior and external jugular veins also pass through this layer. The anterior jugular veins course close to the midline and may assume significant size when the thyroid gland extends to the superior mediastinum, impeding venous drainage. The anterior jugular veins have rare cross-connections in suprasternal space (Space of Burns), which need effective control when the midline is divided. External jugular veins cross obliquely but seldom cause trouble in routine exploration for thyroidectomy (Fig. 4.1). Three pairs of strap muscles (sternothyroid, sternohyoid, and omohyoid) anchor the thyroid gland in the anterior aspect. The sternothyroid muscles are closely applied to each lobe of the thyroid. They are attached to the oblique line of the thyroid cartilage and prevent migration of the enlarged thyroid gland to the anterior aspect of the larynx. But nodules from the superior pole extend the cephaloid towards the submandibular region from behind the sternohyoid muscle close to the carotid sheath on the postero-lateral aspect (Fig. 4.2). Sternocleidomastoid muscles protect the thyroid in the lateral aspect.

The shape and size of the thyroid gland are variable concerning gender and goitrogenic influence, such as iodine deficiency and goitrogens in the diet. Each lobe measures 45–50 mm in length, 12–15 mm in breadth, and 10–12 mm in thickness on sonological assessment. The lobes appear flat or even spherical, and the isthmus

C. G. Nair (✉)
Professor of Surgery, Endocrine Surgery Division, Amrita Institute of Medical Sciences and Research Centre, Kochi, Kerala, India

C. G. Nair, S. J. Abraham (eds.), *Surgical Management of Thyroid and Parathyroid Diseases*, https://doi.org/10.1007/978-981-97-3774-1_4

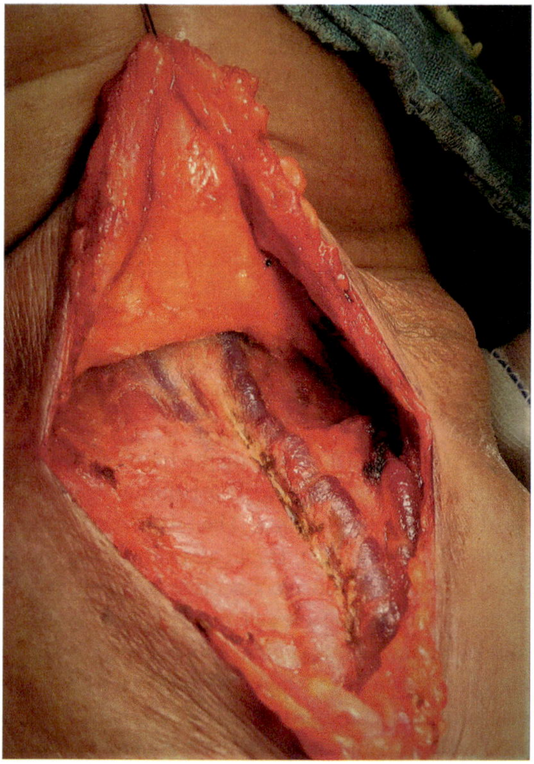

Fig. 4.1 The external jugular vein

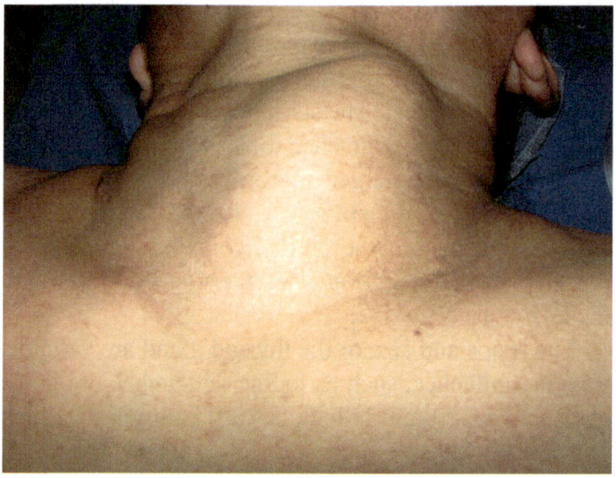

Fig. 4.2 Large volume thyroid nodule from the superior pole

connecting the lobes stretches between the lower third of the lobes or at the lower pole, rendering a U-shaped appearance. The lobe hugs the trachea laterally and extends to the trachea-oesophageal grove. The posterior extent of the lobe reaches the para-spinal muscles. The normal thyroid lobe has a lateral and medial surface, and the posterior rounded border with the carotid sheath structures placed laterally

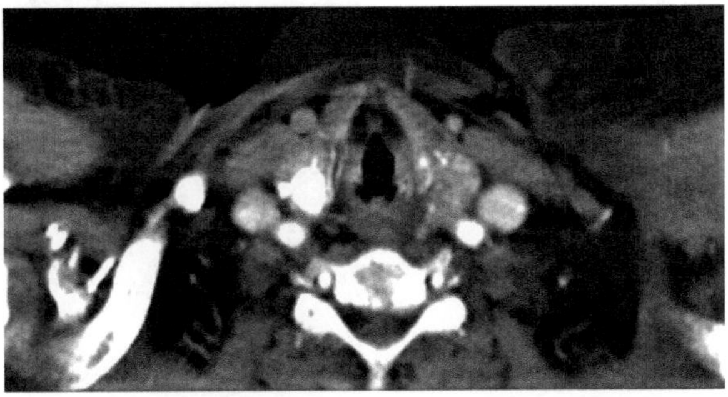

Fig. 4.3 The lobe of the thyroid extends posteriorly displacing the carotid sheath laterally

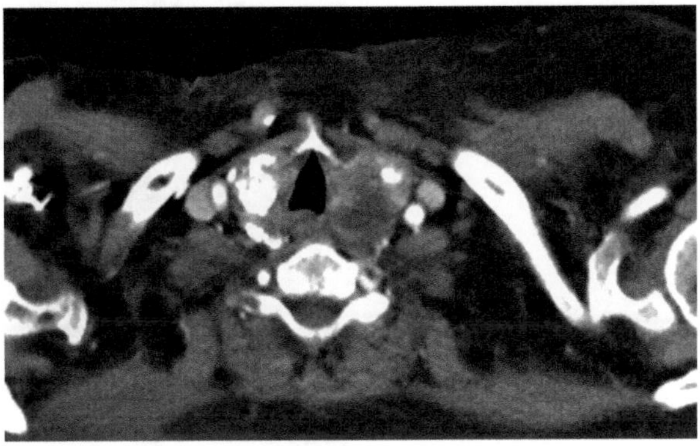

Fig. 4.4 The carotid sheath is displaced

(Fig. 4.3 CT). The posterior border forms the third surface when the lobe enlarges and splays the carotid sheath structures (Fig. 4.4 CT). The common carotid artery lies posterior to the third surface at the thoracic inlet level. Occasionally, the goitre dissects between the trachea and oesophagus and bulges into the tracheal lumen, compromising the airway.

The goitre involving both lobes compresses the trachea from the sides, and the lumen is vertically narrowed. Thyroid nodule compressing the trachea from the anterior aspect produces a horizontal narrowing and can cause weakness of tracheal rings (Figs. 4.5 and 4.6 CT).

The thyroid gland is firmly attached to the larynx by the condensation of pre-tracheal fascia, anchoring the lobes to the thyroid cartilage and the cricoid cartilage. Fibrous bands attach firmly to the lobes and isthmus to the trachea. The caudal extent of the pre-tracheal fascia is open so the enlarged thyroid can extend to the mediastinum.

4.1 Ligament of Berry

The thyroid gland is covered by pre-tracheal fascia and forms the false capsule. Posteriorly, the fascia condenses and forms the posterior suspensory ligament (Ligament of Berry). The ligament is approximately 11.5 mm long (8–14) and

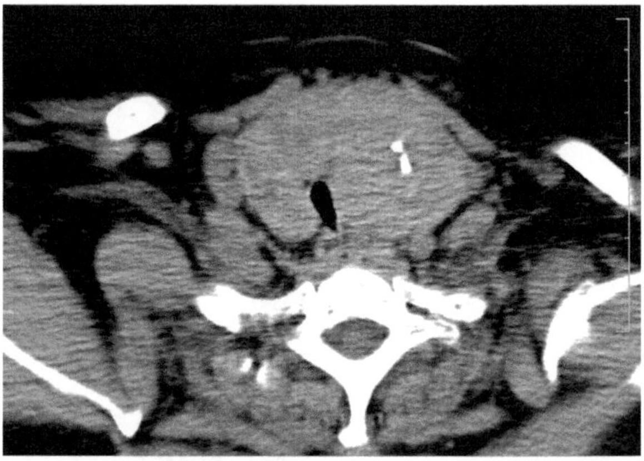

Fig. 4.5 The vertically narrowed trachea

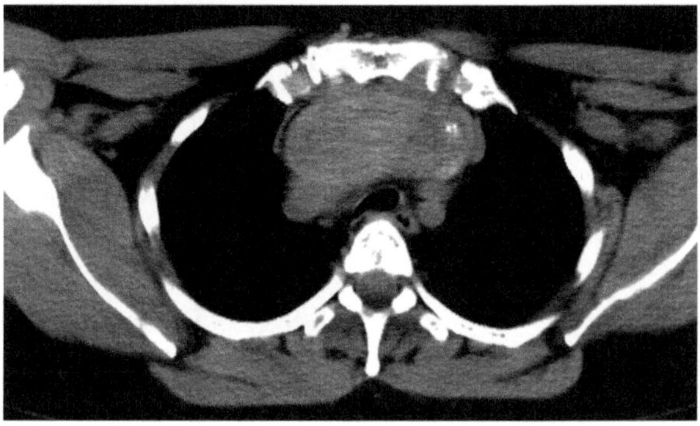

Fig. 4.6 Horizontally compressed trachea

4.4 mm (2–7) wide. It arises from the postero-lateral aspect of the cricoid cartilage and upper tracheal rings. It anchors the posterior surface of the thyroid to the cricoid cartilage and the first, second, and occasionally third tracheal rings (Fig. 4.7).

The ligament is vascular, with the blood supply derived from the Inferior Thyroid Artery (ITA). The ligament is distinctly separable from the true capsule but rarely adhesive. Islets of thyroid tissues are found within the leaflets of the ligament. This anatomic concern questions the completeness of total thyroidectomy in blind capsular dissection to protect the RLN (Fig. 4.8).

The RLN has a variable relation with the ligament coursing posterior to it or mingled within the leaflets of the ligament or perforating it (Fig. 4.9). There is debate in the literature about the exact relationship of the ligament and the RLN, whether it penetrates it or remaining posterior as traditionally regarded [1]. The RLN was most often located superficial to the ligament, with a pooled prevalence estimate of 78.2% of nerves, followed by deep to the ligament in 14.8% [2]. RLN bends sharply towards the terminal portion in about 2% of patients, making it vulnerable to injury (Fig. 4.10). The anterior suspensory ligament anchors the anterior border of the isthmus to the cricoid cartilage and is less fibrous.

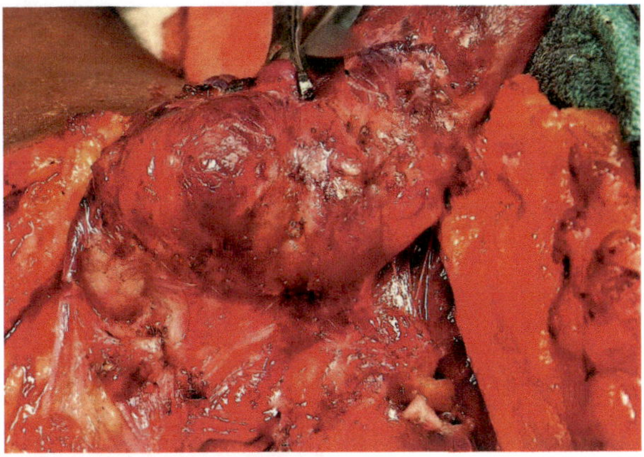

Fig. 4.7 Ligament of Berry, the recurrent laryngeal nerve coursing behind it

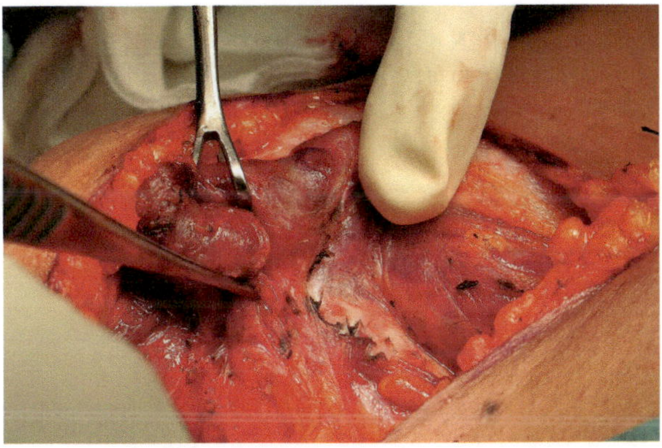

Fig. 4.8 Ligament of Berry with rests of thyroid tissue

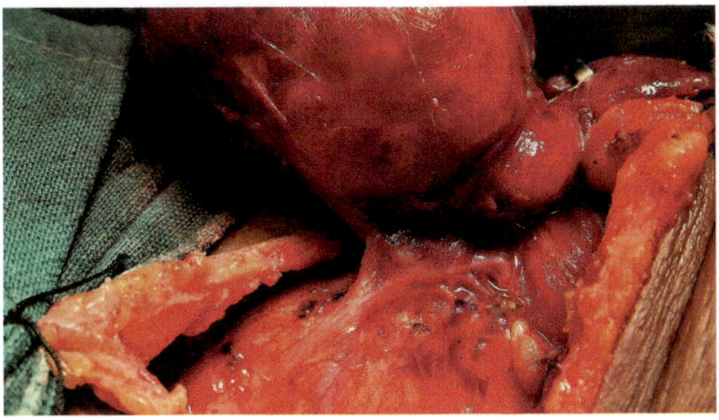

Fig. 4.9 The recurrent laryngeal nerve coursing superficial to the ligament of Berry

Most of the studies of RLN and its relation to ligament are on cadaver dissection so that that operative appearance may differ, especially in patients with cancers, thyroiditis, and recurrence. During the operation, the ligament is exposed when the lobe is medially rotated and held under traction by the assistant modifying the relation (Fig. 4.11).

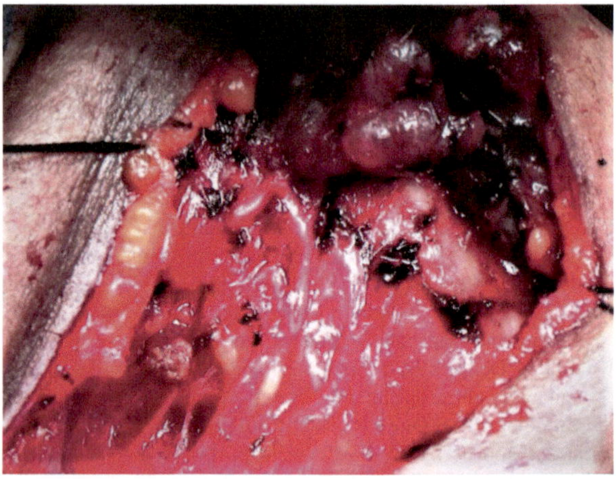

Fig. 4.10 The recurrent laryngeal nerve close to the thyroid near the entry to the larynx

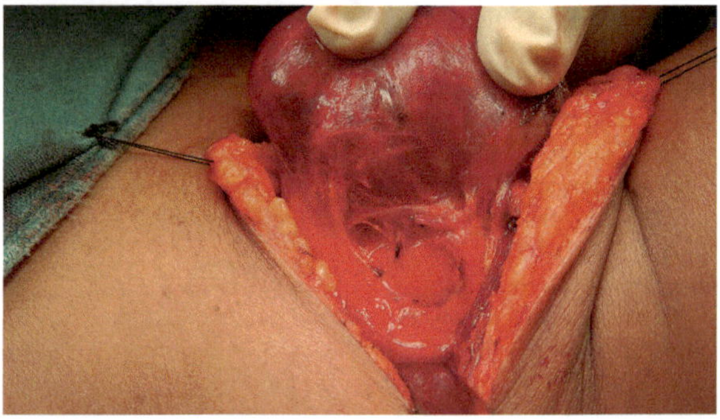

Fig. 4.11 Left RLN coursing posterior to the ligament of Berry

4.2 Ectopic Thyroid

Ectopia occurs when an organ has to migrate to its native location from the site of origin. Embryological thyroid tissue migrates caudally along the midline from the posterior part of the tongue beginning by the 5th week of gestation. The arrest of migration or deviation, of course, is rarely encountered.

Complete failure to migrate results in lingual thyroid, and partial failure leads to ectopic thyroid tissue anywhere in the pathway of descent. Scattered remnants of thyroid tissue are rarely seen in the submandibular triangle, along with the remnants of the thyroglossal tract, thyroid-thymic ligament, and mediastinum (Figs. 4.12, 4.13, 4.14, and 4.15).

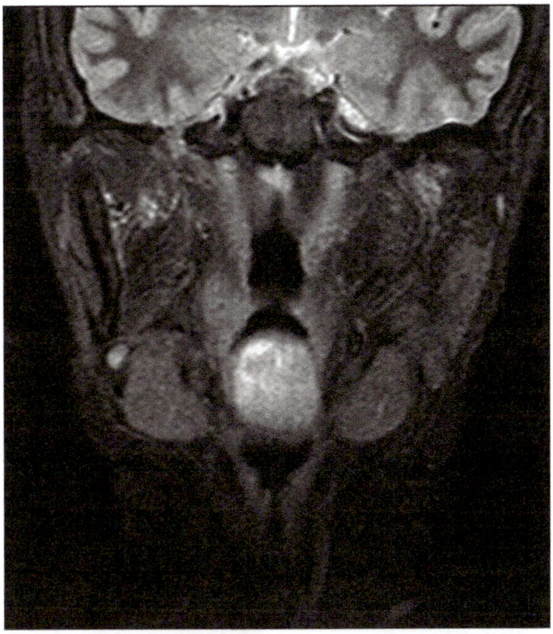

Fig. 4.12 Lingual thyroid

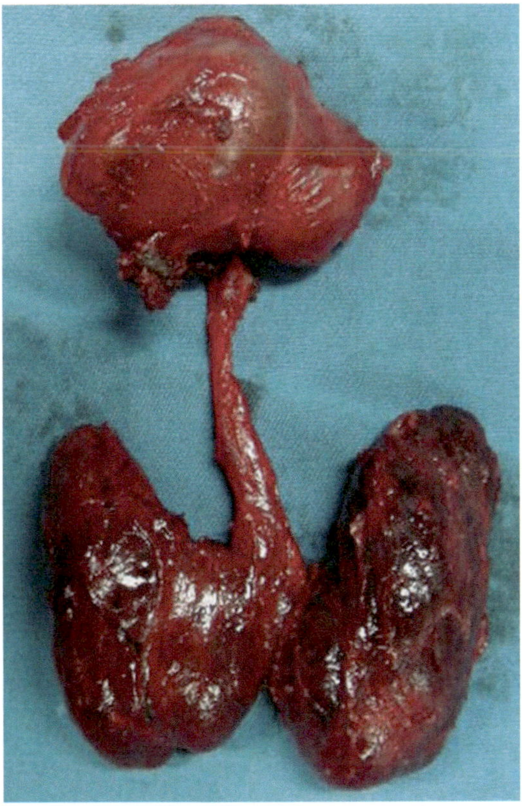

Fig. 4.13 Ectopic thyroid tissue in the thyroglossal tract

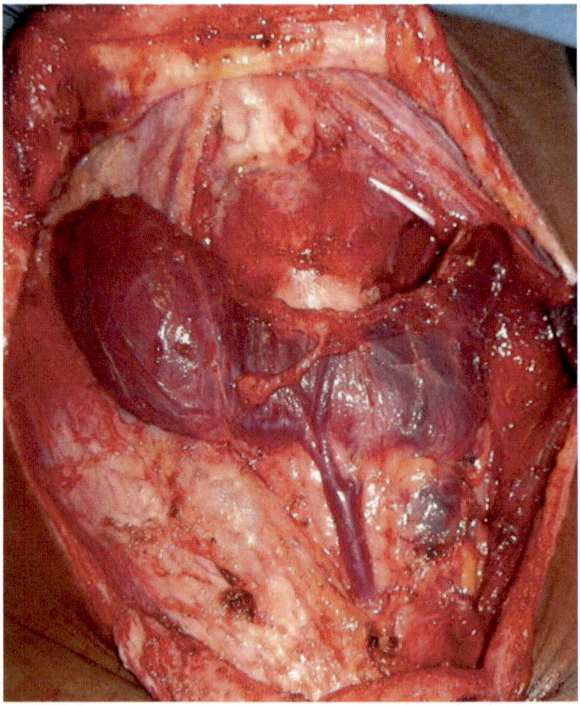

Fig. 4.14 Thyro-thymic ligament rests

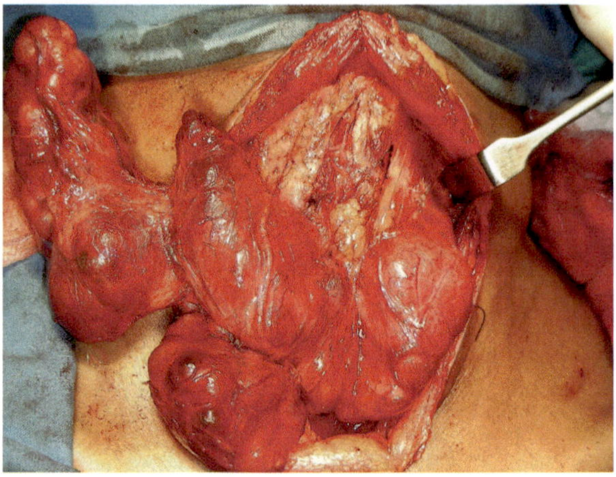

Fig. 4.15 Nodules from tubercle of Zuckerkandl

4.3 Thyro-thymic Rests

Scattered islets of thyroid tissue embedded in soft tissue and thymus are called thyro-thymic rests and are seen in about 50% of patients. The ectopic tissues may retain the connection to the native thyroid and appear as tongue-like protrusions (Grade I). Occasionally, these tissues appear as free islets but with thin fibrous connections (Grade II), and the Grade III are free islets away from the native thyroid. The Grade II and Grade III rests are occasionally mistaken for lymph nodes and are of great significance in Graves' disease and thyroid cancer.

4.4 Pyramidal Lobe and Thyroid Remnants in Thyroglossal Tract

The pyramidal lobe is seen in approximately 50% of patients and represents the terminal portion of the embryological thyroglossal tract. The lobe may be attached to the isthmus's superior border or the medial aspect of the lateral lobes. The pyramidal lobe occasionally harbours a sufficient amount of thyroid tissue and may cause recurrence in Graves' disease or interfere with radioiodine ablation after thyroidectomy for differentiated thyroid cancer (Fig. 4.16).

The tubercle of Zuckerkandl (TZ) is an embryological remembrance on the posterior border of the thyroid lobes. It represents the fusion point of median anlage to the contribution from the ultimobranchial body. This landmark on the middle third of the lobes is a good pointer for identifying the recurrent laryngeal nerve. The tubercle is visible in most occasions (> 80%) and helps the surgeon properly mobilise the lateral aspect of the lobes [3, 4] (Figs. 4.17, 4.18, and 4.19). However, the tubercle is occasionally found in the lower third or the upper third lobe [5].

Based on the size, Pelizzo described a grading system: Grade 0—unrecognisable (11.25%), Grade I—a thickening of the lateral edge (20%), Grade II—1 cm (56.25%), and Grade III—more than 1 cm (12.5%) [3].

The nodule has a variable relation with the recurrent laryngeal nerve; an enlarged nodule may overhang the nerve, hiding it partially and significantly rarely; the nerve may course over the tubercle.

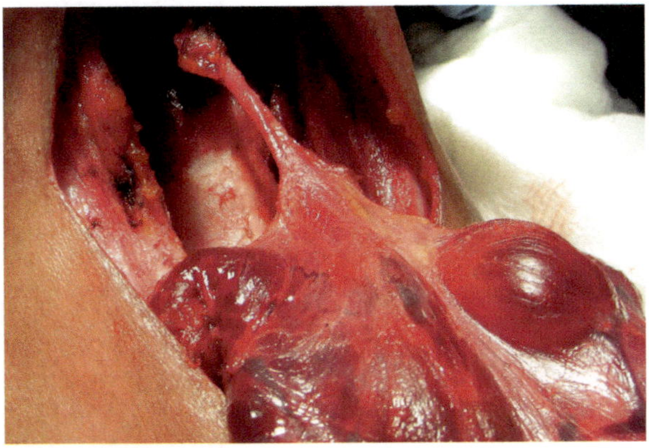

Fig. 4.16 Thyroid tissue in pyramidal lobe

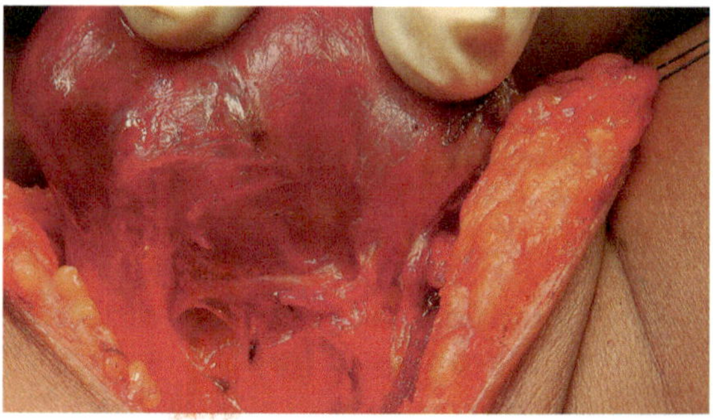

Fig. 4.17 Tubercle of Zuckerkandl and the RLN

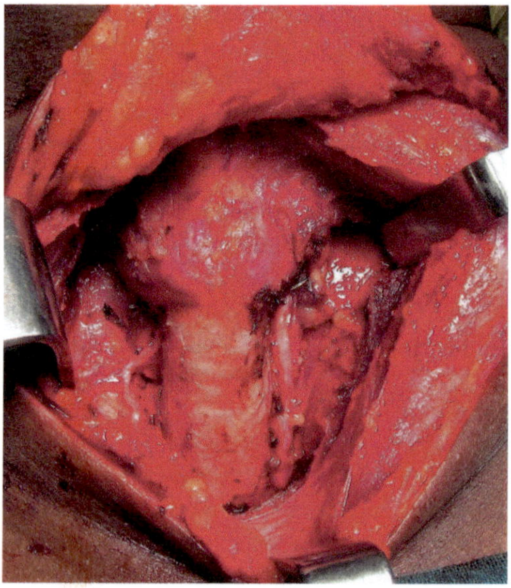

Fig. 4.18 Right and left R LN with different courses

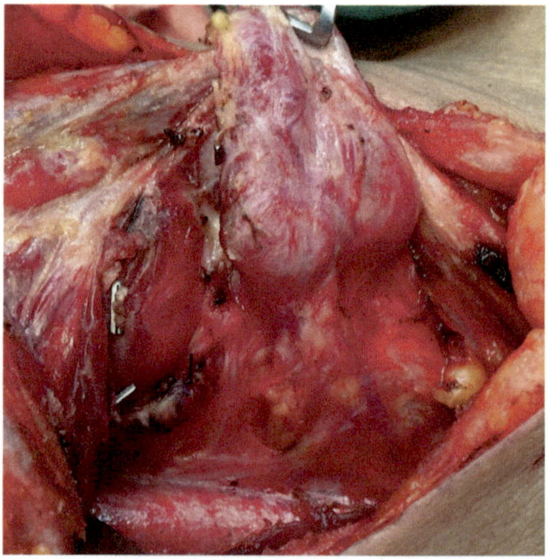

Fig. 4.19 Type 2 non-recurrent RLN

4.5 The Nerves at Risk During Thyroidectomy

The transverse cervical and descending supraclavicular branches of the cervical plexus pierce the deep cervical fascia at the anterior border of the sternomastoid muscle and pass through the sub-platysmal plane. These nerves are in danger when flaps are made.

4.6 The Recurrent Laryngeal Nerve

Recurrent laryngeal nerves (RLN) are crucial in the function of the larynx for phonation and maintaining a normal airway. The nerves transmit the motor fibres of laryngeal muscles and sensory and parasympathetic fibres to laryngeal mucosa below the level of vocal cords. The nerve arises from the vagus nerve at a lower level, ascending to the larynx as it crosses the subclavian artery to reach the tacho-oesophageal grove.

The right and left nerves have different courses to reach the destination. On the left side, it hooks around the aortic arch and takes an oblique course to get the trachea-oesophageal groove after crossing the inferior thyroid artery. The nerve takes a relatively constant course on the left side, passing through the trachea-oesophageal groove towards its entry point to the larynx at the posterior cricothyroid joint (Fig. 4.20). The right RLN is shorter, and its route in the neck is less constant. The right RLN may take a more oblique route and have a shorter course in the trachea-oesophageal groove (Fig. 4.21). Occasionally, the right RLN ascends obliquely over the oesophagus without reaching the groove and gets entry to the larynx directly, making it vulnerable to injury during dissection (Fig. 4.22).

Nonrecurring nerves are rare and almost always seen on the right side and are associated with anomalies of the innominate or subclavian artery and situs inverses. The nonrecurring RLN takes branches of the vagus nerve early and shall run close to the superior thyroid artery (Type 1) or vertically parallel to the inferior thyroid artery (Type 2A) (Fig. 4.23). A scarce type courses along with the trunk of the inferior thyroid artery and mixes with its branches (Type 2B) [4]. But occasionally, regular suitable RLN ascends to the point of entry to the larynx obliquely away from the thyroid gland, almost mimicking a nonrecurrent one (Fig. 4.22).

Berlin and Lahey described the relation between ITA and RLN and its implication in vocal cord paralysis in 1928 [5]. Most RLN courses are behind the inferior thyroid artery's trunk but are rarely seen anterior to the trunk.

The nerve may course anterior to ITA, and the anterior course is more frequent on the right side (35%) than on the left (15%) (Fig. 4.24). Extreme rarely, the RLN courses through the terminal divisions of the inferior thyroid artery and becomes susceptible to injury during capsular dissection (Fig. 4.25). Most anatomical descriptions of RLN were based on cadaver dissection, but the features at operation differ due to changes in gland size and adhesions. The medial rotation of the lobe during operation pulls the nerve more anteriorly [6, 7].

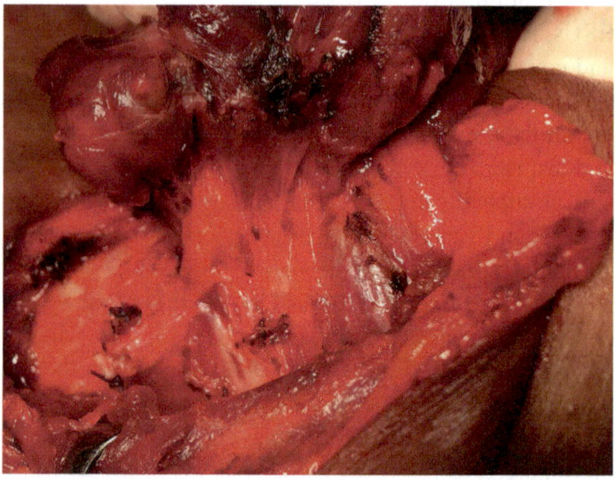

Fig. 4.20 Right RLN away from the thyroid and ligament of Berry

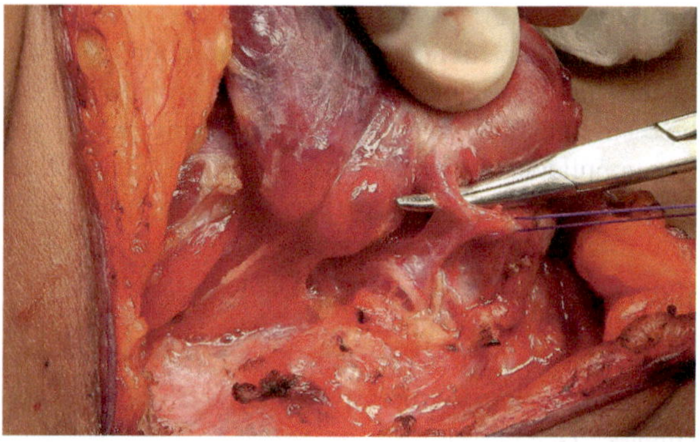

Fig. 4.21 Right RLN coursing superficial to inferior thyroid artery

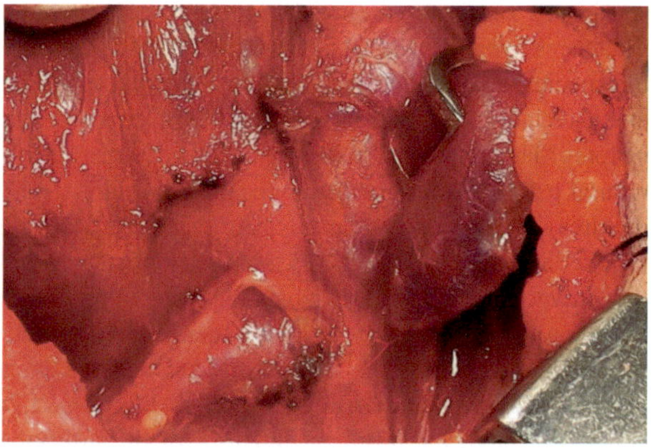

Fig. 4.22 Left RLN coursing on surface of the lobe

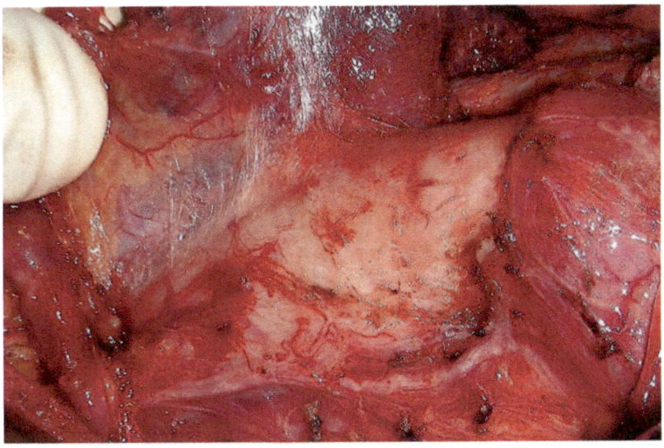

Fig. 4.23 The terminal divisions of RLN

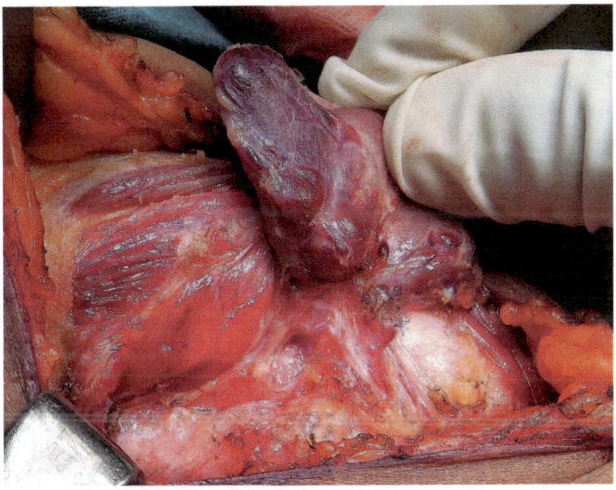

Fig. 4.24 Pre-laryngeal branching of RLN

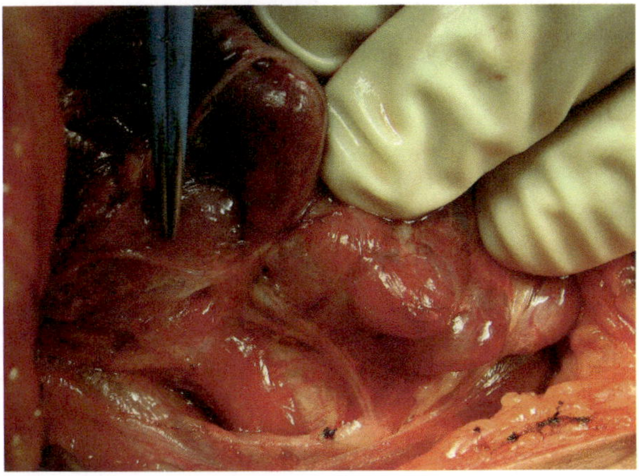

Fig. 4.25 Multiple pre-laryngeal branches

4.7 Branching of RLN

During the surgical procedure, RLN appears as a single trunk until entry to the larynx in approximately 50% of patients (Fig. 4.26). However, the cadaver dissection studies recorded frequent incidences of pre-laryngeal branching [8, 9]. The terminal branches to the laryngeal muscles arise just before entering the larynx (Fig. 4.26). The recorded prevalence of pre-laryngeal branching varies significantly between the cadaveric dissections (73.3%; 95% CI 61.0–84.0) and intraoperative observation (39.2%; 95% CI 29.0–49.9) studies. However, the pooled data did not differ significantly in the prevalence based on the patient's sex or the side of the nerve [8, 9].

Bifurcations are relatively common, but trifurcations and multiple divisions are rare. Branching of RLN is occasional before the nerve meets the RLN and is more frequent in terminal 1–2 cm (Figs. 4.27 and 4.28).

Electrophysiological studies during surgical procedures reported the presence of a positive motor signal in the anterior and posterior branches. However, about 99.9% of the positive motor signals were obtained from the anterior branches and infrequently from the posterior branches [10, 11]. The anterior nerve is at risk during dissection, especially when it crosses Berry's ligament. The nerve is close to the posterior aspect of the lobe and should be cautiously dissected when the ligament harbours thyroid tissues. A few advised intraoperative nerve monitoring, but a recent metanalysis failed to establish the superiority of nerve monitoring over intraoperative localisation [12].

During the surgical procedure, the location of anatomical landmarks such as the inferior thyroid artery, ligament of Berry, tracheoesophageal groove, or tubercle of Zuckerkandl may help to identify the RLN. However, these landmarks are disturbed by asymmetrical enlargement with nodules, enlarged central compartment lymph nodes, and malignant infiltration. Operative manures like an excessive retraction or

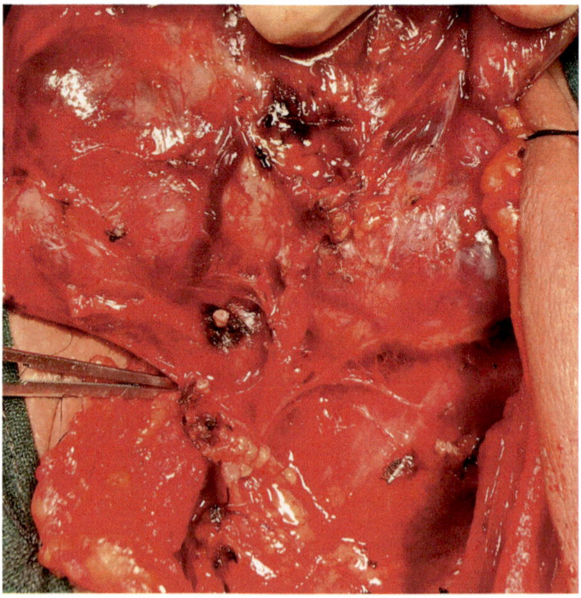

Fig. 4.26 Left RLN, the anterior pre-laryngeal branch coursing on the surface of the lobe

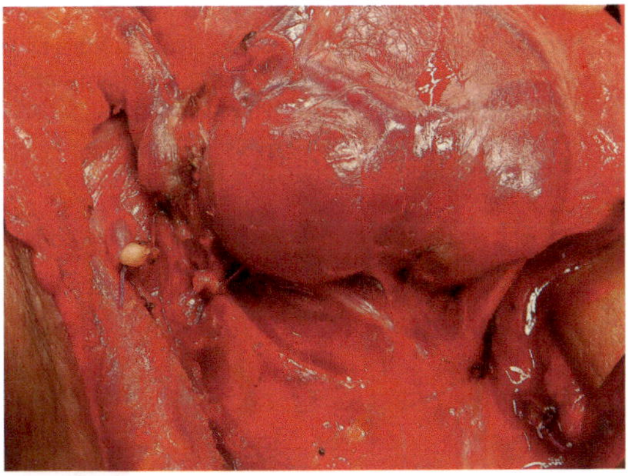

Fig. 4.27 Right RLN-Early bifurcation

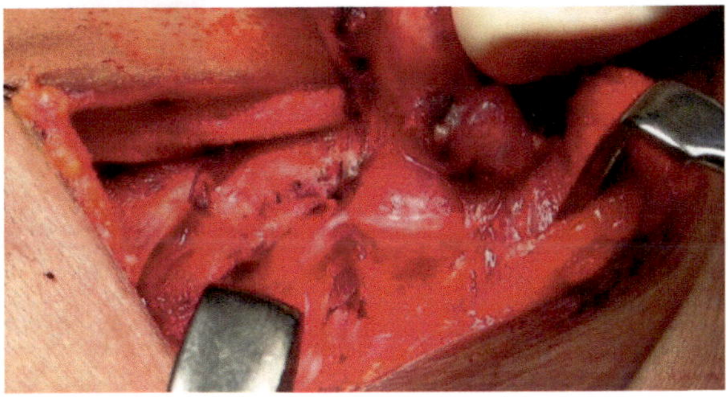

Fig. 4.28 Left RLN coursing on the surface of nodule of tubercle of Zuckerkandl

medial rotation of lobes modify the described anatomy. The tubercle of Zuckerkandl is a relatively stable landmark for RLN during thyroidectomy, with nerve coursing behind it on most occasions. Extreme rarely, the nerve could be lifted to its surface by a nodule from the tubercle (Figs. 4.30 and 4.31). The RLN has a variable relation with the ligament of Berry and was discussed earlier in detail.

4.8 External Branch of Superior Laryngeal Nerve (EBSLN)

The superior laryngeal nerve leaves the vagal trunk above the level of carotid artery bifurcation, and the internal division pierces the thyrohyoid membrane to reach the larynx. The external division (EBSLN) descends and crosses the superior thyroid artery at the variable level to reach the cricothyroid muscle. Based on the relation with the superior thyroid artery, Cernea et al. described three types (Table 4.1) [13]. Kierner et al. modified the Type 2 B relationship based on the anterior or posterior nerve course to the superior thyroid vessels [14] (Figs.4.29, 4.30, 4.31, 4.32, 4.33, and 4.34).

Table 4.1 Various classifications of EBSLN

Type 1: The nerve crosses STA >1 cm above the upper pole.
Type 2A: The nerve crosses STA <1 cm above the upper pole of the thyroid.
Type 2B: The nerve crosses STA under cover of the upper pole of the thyroid.

Symmetric contraction of the cricothyroid muscles causes lengthening and thinning of vocal cords by raising the anterior cricoid cartilages. Paralysis of the cricothyroid muscle reduces the highest obtainable fundamental frequency and decreases high vocal projection [15]. Reports show a connection from the EBSLN to the mid-portion of the thyroarytenoid muscle, which may assist in the adduction of the vocal fold [16]. Further, a communication branch between RLN and EBSLN was observed in students, ranging from 25 to 77.3% [17, 18]. The function of this communication is uncertain and considered to contribute to sensory distribution [19]

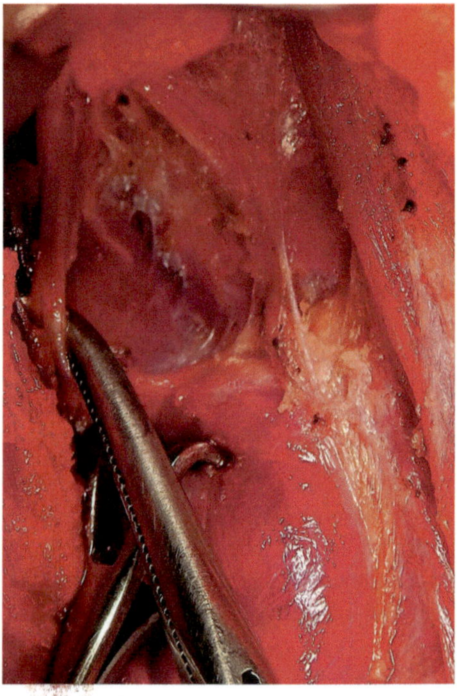

Fig. 4.29 Type 1 EBSLN

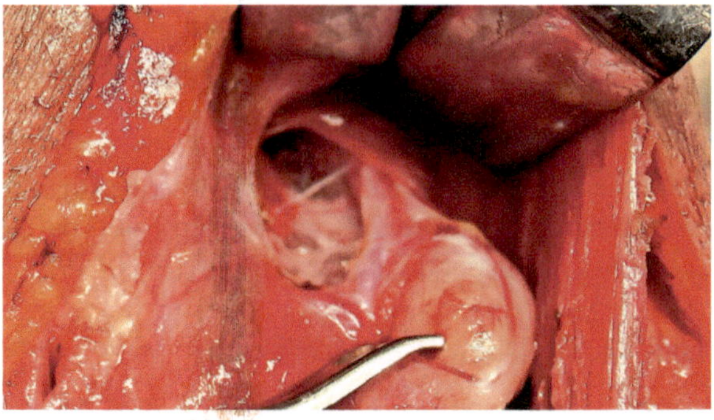

Fig. 4.30 Type 2 EBSLN

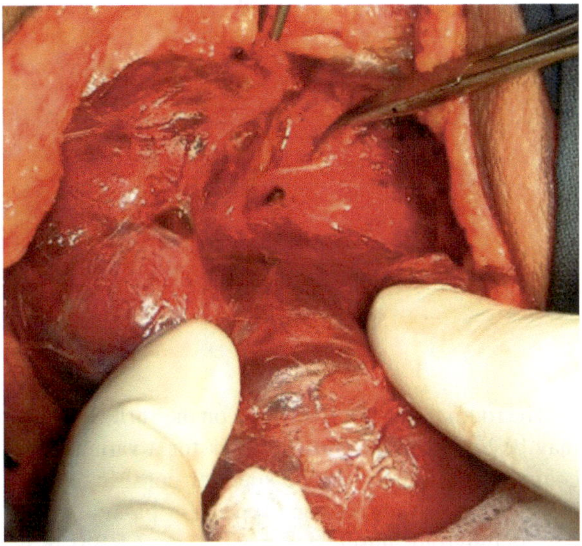

Fig. 4.31 Type 3 EBSLN

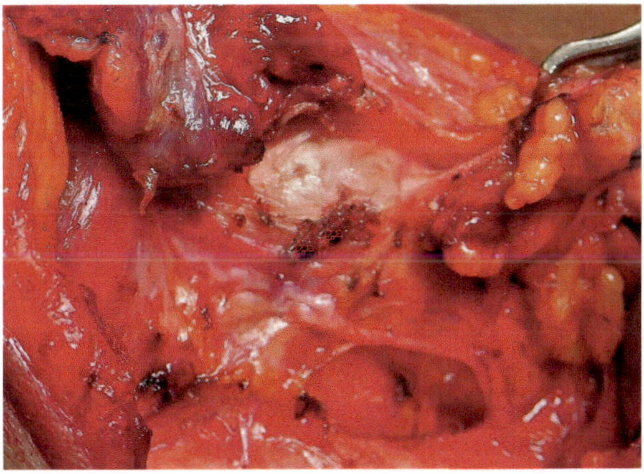

Fig. 4.32 Galen's anastomosis

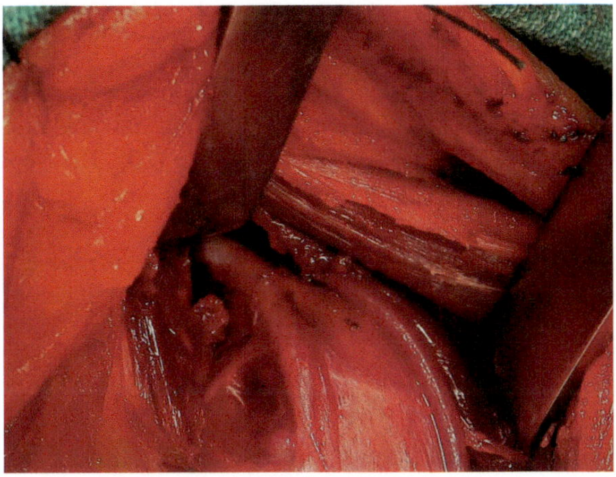

Fig. 4.33 Type 2, EBSLN coursing behind the superior thyroid vessels

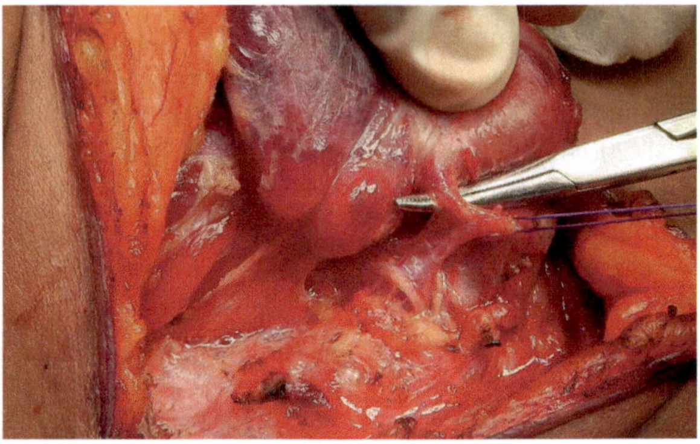

Fig. 4.34 RLN coursing superficial to the inferior thyroid artery

The routine route of EBSLN is on the surface of superior constrictor muscles and may be buried in the muscle fibres for a variable part of its course [14]. EBSLN courses superficially on the superior constrictor muscle (Type 1), penetrates the muscle at the lower portion (Type 2) or passes through the fibres of SCM towards the cricothyroid muscle (Type 3). Type 3 EBSLN is not visible in the cricothyroid space.

Kierner Classification

Type 1: The nerve crosses STA >1 cm above the upper pole of the thyroid.
Type 2: The nerve crosses STA <1 cm above the upper pole of the thyroid.
Type 3: Crosses STA under cover of the upper pole of the thyroid.
Type 4: Descends dorsal to the artery and crosses STA branches immediately above the upper pole of the thyroid.

Friedman has described three variants of the EBSLN as detailed below:

Type 1: The nerve runs superficial to the inferior constrictor muscle.
Type 2: The nerve penetrates the lower part of the inferior constrictor muscle.
Type 3: The nerve runs deep into the inferior constrictor muscle.

4.9 Blood Supply

The thyroid gland is very rich in blood supply, receiving a mean blood flow of 18.3 mL/min (5.8–29.2) in the euthyroid state and increasing to a mean of 73 mL/min (30–140) in the hyperthyroid state [20]. The Superior Thyroid Artery (STA) and Inferior Thyroid Artery (ITA) are significant arteries of surgical significance.

The STA is a relatively constant source of blood supply to the thyroid and is traditionally considered a branch of the external carotid artery. Rarely, it may take

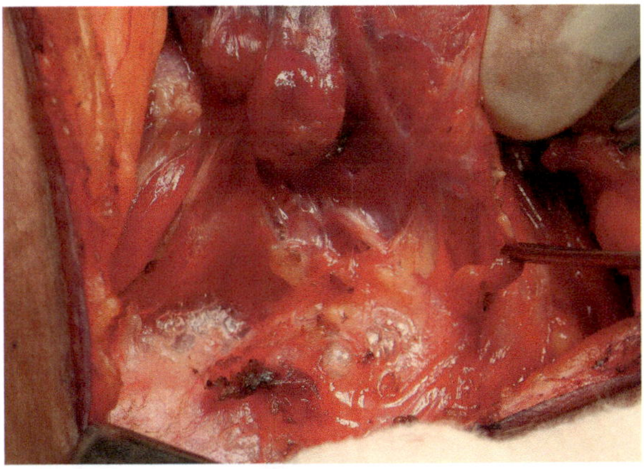

Fig. 4.35 The superior and inferior parathyroid glands right side

the origin from a common carotid at the bifurcation or as a common trunk with a lingual artery or facial artery. The superior thyroid artery is the primary source of blood supply to the thyroid gland but also gives branches to the adjacent muscles and skin. The artery deseeds from its origin on the lateral aspect of the larynx under cover of the superior belly of the Omo-hyoid muscle, giving laryngeal and muscular branches. STA terminates, giving anterior and posterior glandular branches on 90% of occasions, but a lateral branch is seen rarely (Fig. 4.35). The terminal branches arise approximately 2 cm away from the superior pole of the gland, and the anterior branches are anastomoses, forming a supra isthmic arch. The supra isthmic plexus becomes a collateral pathway in unilateral carotid obstruction. Branches supplying thyroid glandular tissue enter directly or course on the surface before penetrating the capsule. The posterior branch anastomoses with the inferior thyroid artery, forming a longitudinal anastomotic arch. The superior parathyroid gland may receive blood from the longitudinal anastomotic arch.

The variable relation between the STA and EBSLN is discussed in detail earlier. Superior thyroid veins are relatively constant and receive venous drainage from the larynx. The corresponding veins accompany the artery and drain directly to the internal jugular vein or indirectly after joining the common facial vein.

4.10 Inferior Thyroid Artery (ITA) (Fig. 4.36)

Approximately 80% of ITA originates from the Thyrocervical trunk; the other sources of origin are the common carotid, subclavian, and vertebral arteries. ITA may be absent in 1–6% and is found to be more constant on the right side [21]. The artery courses superiorly and turns medially at the sixth cervical transverse process level to reach the posterior border of the gland after breaking down into two to three

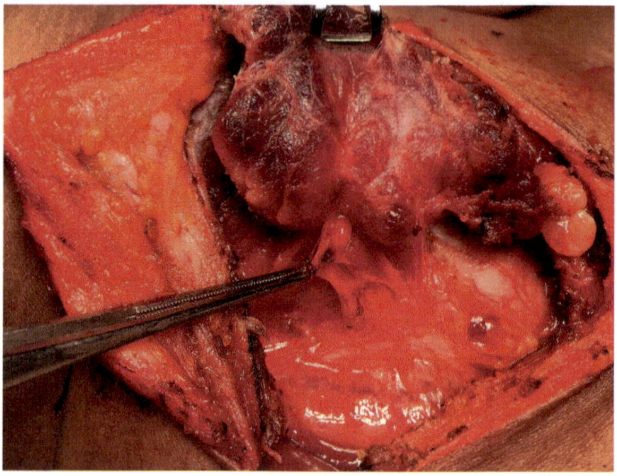

Fig. 4.36 The superior parathyroid gland inside the false capsule of thyroid

terminal branches (medial, inferior, and posterior). ITA is considered the prime source of blood supply to parathyroid glands. Sequential occlusion of superior and inferior thyroid vessels and flow measurement with Laser Doppler Flowmetry established ITA as the primary source of parathyroid blood supply [22]. Primarily, the parathyroid receives one artery and occasionally gets an additional artery. Inferior parathyroid glands receive their arterial supply from the ITA; the artery arises from the trunk or one of the terminal divisions, more commonly from the lower division. During the division of terminal branches of ITA, it is always advisable to inspect the parathyroid vessel closely.

The superior parathyroid glands have a relatively variable source of blood supply, the arterial twig arising from the ITA or the longitudinal retro-lobar anastomosis between ITA and STA. During thyroidectomy, STA has to be ligated so the anastomotic arch receives blood from the ITA and preserving the arch is of paramount significance for parathyroid perfusion [23]. A vein does not accompany the inferior thyroid artery but forms a plexus below the isthmus.

The venous drainage of the thyroid gland is complex, with many named and unnamed veins. Middle thyroid veins are standard on the right side but less frequently seen on the left side. This short, stumpy vein assumes a large size in high vascular thyroid as in hyperthyroidism and drains directly to the internal jugular vein. This vein merits careful handling since injury leads to heavy bleeding. Less frequently, another vein called the third vein, is found inferior to the middle thyroid vein. Close to the superior pole of the lobe on the lateral aspects, occasionally, a single trunk or multiple small veins are found draining directly to the internal jugular vein. The inferior thyroid veins are a plexus of veins or one or two trunks almost arising from the lower pole and course on the anterior aspect of the trachea. These veins form a single trunk and course through the remnants of the cervical thymus to drain into the innominate vein. These veins are better divided close to the thyroid gland to prevent thermal injury to the inferior parathyroid gland and its blood supply (Fig. 4.37).

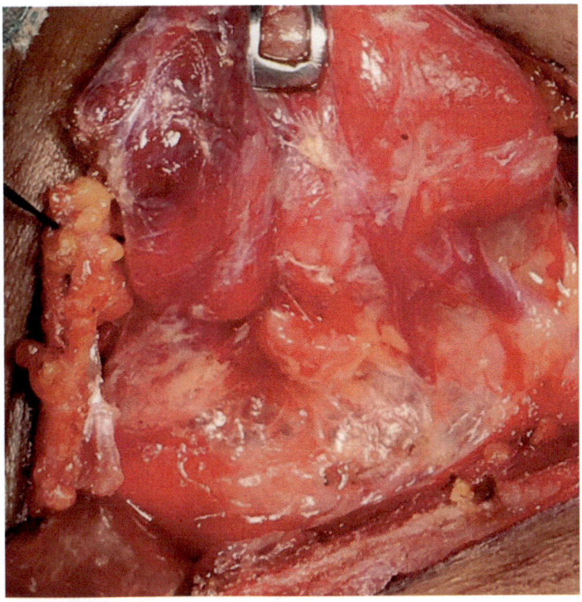

Fig. 4.37 Middle thyroid vein and third vein

4.11 Parathyroid Glands

The parathyroid glands are usually four in number and control the calcium homeostasis. These tiny structures, usually four in number, have variable relations to the thyroid glands and are of paramount significance in neck surgical procedures. The loss of function of parathyroid glands leads to severe morbidity and requires costly lifelong dependence on supplements.

Parathyroid glands are identified by their characteristic brown colour in fat, like a small chocolate fragment embedded in butter and roughly oval. The normal gland seldom measures more than a centimetre. The superior parathyroid glands, the fourth parathyroid, indicating their embryological origin from the fourth pharyngeal arch, are more constant in position. They are seen close to the posterior border of the upper third of the thyroid lobes, closely related to the terminal portion of RLN. They derive the blood supply directly from the inferior thyroid artery or the posterior anastomotic plexus between the superior and inferior thyroid arteries (Fig. 4.38).

The inferior parathyroid glands develop from the third pharyngeal pouch along with the thymus and descend along with the thymus to occupy their usual position. They are less stable in position and are mostly seen a centimetre or two away from the inferior thyroid artery. They are more likely to occupy ectopic locations in the mediastinum. The glands receive arterial twigs directly from the ITA or its divisions. Ectopic locations are mediastinum, within the false capsule of the thyroid gland, intrathyroidal, and carotid sheath (Fig. 4.39).

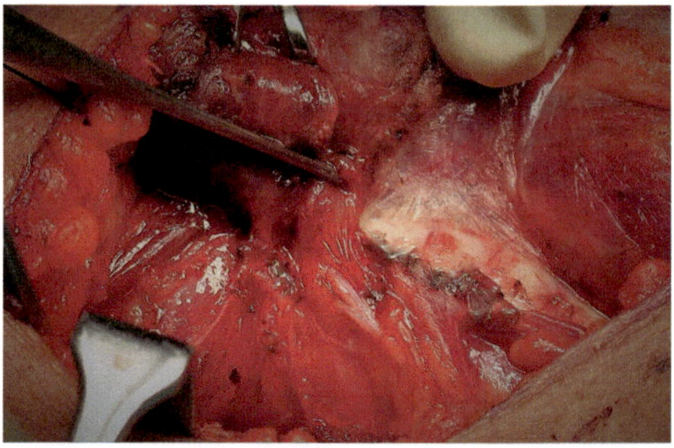

Fig. 4.38 Superior parathyroid and the ligament of Berry

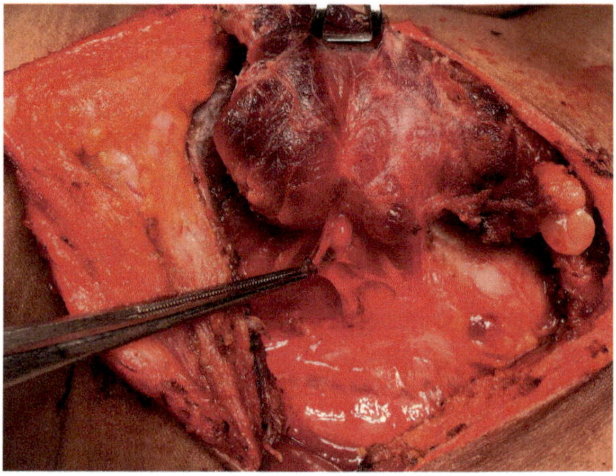

Fig. 4.39 Superior and inferior parathyroid glands

4.12 Lymphatic Drainage

The thyroid gland has a rich network of lymphatic channels and shows multidirectional flow. Four distinct drainage patterns are recognised: median superior drainage, median inferior drainage, right/left lateral drainage, and posterior drainage (Holinshed drainage pattern) [24, 25].

The median superior channels may be connected to the pre-laryngeal nodal station or drain directly to the jugulo-digastric station. The right and left lateral channels drain into para-tracheal nodes or follow superior or inferior thyroid vessels. The median inferior channels arise from the lower border of the isthmus and medial aspect of the lower pole of the thyroid end in pre-tracheal, para-tracheal, and subclavian nodes.

The pattern of lymph nodes affected by thyroid cancers is to pre-laryngeal, paratracheal, or pre-tracheal nodes and then to the lateral deep cervical chain. However, due to the bizarre pattern of lymphatic channels, skipping metastases to lateral nodal stations is not uncommon.

4.13 Physiology of Thyroid Gland

The thyroid gland is enclosed within a false capsule derived from the pre-tracheal fascia and a true capsule. The thyroid gland is divided into many lobules separated by septae extending from the fibroblastic true capsule. Each lobule contains multiple follicles. Follicles are functional and structural units of the thyroid gland lined by cuboidal cells called the follicular cells resting on the basement membrane. During development, parafollicular cells or C-cells are derived from the neural crest cells reaching the thyroid through the ultimobranchial body. Parafollicular cells are placed between the follicular cells, and the cells seldom reach the lumen of follicles and do not contribute to the normal functioning of the thyroid [26–28].

The central lumen of follicles contains a colloid composed of thyroglobulin. Thyroglobulin is a glycoprotein uniquely synthesised by the endoplasmic reticulum of follicular cells and stored in the lumen of follicles. The space between follicles is filled by connective tissue stroma, and the blood vessels, nerves, and lymphatics traverse the septae before reaching the follicles.

The thyroid gland produces approximately 100 μg of thyroxine in 24 h, 80–90% of which are tetraiodothyronine and the rest triiodothyronine. Thyroid hormone synthesis differs from other endocrine glands since most synthesis steps are not intracellular. The essential substrate required for synthesis is iodine, and the availability of this is a strong determinant of thyroid dysfunction diseases.

An average uptake of 100–150 μg/day is adequate for normal regular synthesis of thyroxine. Thyroid follicular cells concentrate approximately 20% iodine reaching the gland and can store 20–50 times higher than serum concentration [29]. There is considerable iodine uptake in salivary glands, gastric mucosa, and lactating breasts. The former two locations share standard embryological derivation from foregut mucosa. Lactating breasts concentrate iodine and excrete it through milk [30]. These uptakes gain significance when the radioactive form of iodine is used for therapeutic purposes.

Iodine uptake of follicular cells (thyrocytes) is an active energy-requiring process. A protein called sodium/iodide symporter (NIS) mediates this dynamic process on the basolateral plasma membrane of thyrocytes. The iodine pool in the thyrocytes is a mixture of iodine brought in by NIS and by deiodination of iodinated thyronine.

Iodine entering thyrocytes reaches the colloid in a short time for further oxidation. The iodine moieties diffuse towards the apical end of the cells and to colloid facilitated by an anion exchange protein called pendrin [31]. Iodine is oxidised, organified and attached to free tyrosine moieties in thyroglobulin. This process is continuously catalysed by thyroperoxidase in the presence of H_2O_2. The H_2O_2 is generated under dual oxidase 2 (DUOX 2) and is essential for iodine oxidation. The pathways responsible for H_2O_2 production at the apical plasma membrane were known long before [32]. DUOX 1 and 2 genes regulate DUOX expression, and mutations disrupt hormone synthesis, resulting in Dyshormonogenesis. Oxidation iodine produces monoiodotyrosine and diiodotyrosine, and the iodinated moieties coupled with the neighbouring ones form tetraiodothyronines or triiodothyronines. TPO catalyses the final step of hormone synthesis also.

The iodothyronines are stored in colloid and released to circulation by another series of processes governed by TSH. Thyroglobulin containing the iodinated tyrosine is taken into vesicles on the cell membrane and finally enters the follicular cells by a process of endocytosis similar to phagocytosis. Thyroglobulin remains in the cell as free radicles or in combination with receptor proteins and later undergoes hydrolysis in lysosomal compartments, releasing free hormones and thyroglobulin residues. The mechanism of hormone release to the bloodstream is unclear but thought to be by simple diffusion. A small but significant amount of free thyroglobulin also leaks out to the bloodstream, gaining significance in the follow-up of DTC patients.

4.13.1 Transport of Hormones in the Blood

Lipophilic Thyroid Hormones are transported in the bloodstream with proteins, mainly to the thyroxine-binding globulin (TBG) and prealbumin (transthyretin). A fraction of thyroid hormone (~0.2%) remains free in the bloodstream and is biologically active. In specific locations, the inactive T4 is converted to active T3 by a group of deiodinase enzymes, Type I, II, and III. The differential presence of the deiodinase enzyme is also a controlling factor of hormonal function.

Thyroid hormones are metabolised in the liver by sulfation and glucuronidation, whereby they are converted to hydrophilic and excreted through bile to the intestine. The sulfation pathway is irreversible, and sulfated iodothyronines are excreted. However, the glucuronides are hydrolysed by bacterial hydroxylases and reabsorbed, leading to enterohepatic circulation, which gains significance in Graves' disease.

4.13.2 Regulation

The hypothalamic—Pituitary—thyroid axis is the master control of the thyroxine-secreting system. Both the hypothalamus and pituitary respond to circulating T4, which is converted to T3 by Type II deiodinase and releases thyrotropin-releasing hormone (TRH) and TSH, respectively. Local conversion of T4 to T3 induces negative feedback whereby the decreased concentration of T3 stimulates the secretion of TRH and TSH. The hypothalamus plays a significant role in the circadian rhythm of hormone production and release. TSH enhances Na/I symporter and further pathways of synthesis and release of hormones from thyroglobulin.

4.13.3 Actions

Tetraiodothyronine (T4) is the inactive precursor and is cleaved to active forms 3, 5, and 3-triiodothyronine by deiodinase enzymes in specific target cells. The cleavage results in both functional and inactive rT3, which is degraded and added to the iodine reserve.

Thyroid hormone is essential for the normal development of tissues and the regulation of metabolic pathways. The actions are imparted through thyroid hormone receptors (TR) and are expressed in alpha and beta isoforms. There is differential expression of these isoforms in tissues, which probably determines the tissue-specific action of thyroid hormone. TR @ receptors are predominantly in the brain, skeletal muscles, and heart. TR beta receptors have three splice products and are distributed widely, but beta-3 is expressed in the kidneys, liver, and lungs.

Thyroid hormone is a crucial regulator of Basal metabolic rate (BMR), but the pathways are not established. The hormone increases lipid, glucose, and protein metabolic cycles, but their contribution to increasing BMR is limited. TH maintains the balanced state of metabolism of lipids, carbohydrates, and proteins in normal ranges of serum levels. Higher levels induce protein catabolism, gluconeogenesis, glucose oxidation, and lipolysis.

TH enhances the effects of catecholamines and leads to overexpression of beta-receptors. TH stimulates respiratory centres and increases respiratory rate and efforts. In children, the thyroid hormone acts synergistically with growth hormone and is required for brain maturation.

4.14 Parathyroid Glands; Histology and Function

Parathyroid glands regulate calcium homeostasis, and the control is mediated through the bones, gastrointestinal tract, and kidneys. Four glands are distributed near the thyroid glands, originating from the third and fourth pharyngeal arch. They are less than 10 mm in size and have bean-like shapes, weighing less than 40 mg. Parathyroid glands share the blood supply with the thyroid gland. The characteristic appearance of the gland is a bead of chocolate embedded in the butter, and trained eyes differentiate them from lymph nodes.

The superior parathyroid glands are derived from the third pharyngeal pouch. They are placed in close contact with the upper third of the posterior border of each lobe near the entry of the recurrent laryngeal nerve to the larynx. They are relatively constant in position but necessitate careful dissection at the level of the ligament of Berry. Mostly, inferior thyroid arteries are the source of blood supply but occasionally receive from the posterior anastomotic plexus or the superior thyroid artery.

Inferior glands develop from the third arch along with the thymus and are mostly wanderers since the position is not constant. They are commonly seen in one centimetre near the lower poles of the thyroid lobes but are infrequently located in the mediastinum or carotid sheath. They receive the blood vessels from the inferior thyroid arteries. Inferior parathyroid glands are mistaken for lymph nodes and thyro-thymic rests.

Parathyroid glands comprise Chief cells, adipose cells, and scattered clusters of oxyphil cells. Chief cells are the primary secretory cells, and when these cells are active, many dense, irregularly shaped secretory granules are visible within the cytoplasm on electron microscopy. The active ingredient of parathyroid extract was isolated by Collip in 1925 [33]. Rasmussen and Craig isolated and purified the parathyroid hormone and defined its polypeptide structure in 1962 [34]. The cellular components of parathyroid glands are chief cells, adipocytes and clusters of oxyphil cells scattered throughout the stroma. Water-clear cells are seen scantly. Chief cells are rich in mitochondria, and in the active phase, secretory granules, large Golgi complexes, and free ribosomes are visible clearly in electron microscopy [35]. Oxyphil cells are larger, rich in mitochondria, and seen in humans and certain animals. They are more frequent in old age but are metabolically active and possess a higher amount of oxidative and hydrolytic enzymes than chief cells [35].

4.15 Physiology of Parathyroid Glands

The Chief cells constitute the main bulk of functioning cells engaged in parathyroid hormone synthesis and play a key role in calcium homeostasis. The calcium-sensing receptors are sensitive to extracellular calcium and exert a negative feedback control on parathyroid hormone synthesis and release.

Oxyphil cells are seen in singles or small clusters dispersed among the chief cells. They are larger in size and rich in mitochondria. They were considered inactive and derived from chief cells. Chief cell proliferation occurs during hypocalcaemia, and the inessential excess cells, after cessation of the stimulus, are converted to oxyphil cells since the chief cells do not undergo apoptosis. However, whether increased metabolic activity in oxyphil cells reflects PTH secretion is unclear [36, 37].

The third cell type is the rare water-clear cell, which possesses an oval or round nucleus, and the cytoplasm is filled with membrane-limited vacuoles. The clear cells are more with ageing and are not influenced by the change of serum PTH levels [37].

Parathyroid hormone is a polypeptide that is essentially synthesised by chief cells as a 115 amino acid chain but undergoes two-step cleavages to form active parathyroid hormone comprised of 84 amino acids. The hormone is stored and secreted as an active form but rapidly undergoes disintegration in the liver and kidney. The intact PTH has a very short half-life of 2–4 min, and it is cleaved into active amino- and inactive carboxyl-terminal fragments that are then cleared by the kidney. The carboxyl-terminal fragments have a five to ten-times longer half-life.

Extracellular calcium, phosphate, calcitriol, and fibroblast growth factor 23 (FGF23) regulate PTH synthesis and secretion from parathyroid glands. Extracellular calcium is found to have an inverse-sigmoidal curve in relation to PTH. The negative feedback mechanism is mediated through Calcium-sensing sensing receptors (Ca SR) in parathyroid cells. High extracellular calcium halts the PTH synthesis and secretion, and low level releases the inhibition. The threshold level of ionised calcium has a narrow range, and a swing of 0.1 mg/dL alters PTH secretion significantly. Persistent lowering of ionic calcium induces cellular hyperplasia of the parathyroid [38].

Hyperphosphatemia stimulates parathyroid cells to secrete PTH, but the exact pathway is still uncertain. A direct role of phosphate in inhibiting the Ca SR activity via non-competitive antagonism has been suggested, but subtle changes do not induce PTH secretion [37]. Parathyroid cells express vitamin D receptors, and calcitriol inhibits PTH synthesis by binding to the vitamin D receptor. Calcitriol also inhibits parathyroid cell proliferation [39].

Fibroblast growth factor-23 (FGF23) is a glycoprotein produced in the bone by osteoblasts and osteocytes under physiological circumstances. On mineral metabolism, FGF23 exerts a suppressive effect on phosphate reabsorption from the urine. In addition, FGF23 suppresses calcitriol synthesis in the kidney and exerts a catabolic stimulant effect [40]. In addition to its phosphaturic action, FGF23 directly acts on the parathyroid gland, inhibiting PTH synthesis and secretion.

4.16 Actions

Parathyroid hormone is the critical factor in calcium homeostasis. PTH mobilises calcium from the bone, conserves calcium in the kidneys, and facilitates absorption in the intestine.

The bone is the rich source of calcium in the body and is constantly in the process of remodelling. There is an equilibrium in the bone resorption and new bone formation under osteoblastic and osteoclastic activities, respectively. Bone remodelling is a coupled process of resorption and formation. PTH targets osteoblasts and osteocytes directly and osteoclasts indirectly to enhance bone remodelling. The receptor activator of nuclear factor-kappaB ligand (RANKL)/RANK/osteoprotegerin (OPG) system and its role in regulating bone resorption [41]. PTH stimulation increases the RANKL/OPG ratio, favouring osteoclast activity. The chronic activity of PTH favours excessive osteoclastic activity, resulting in bone loss.

The kidney plays a significant role in the normal homeostasis of mineral metabolism. Most of the filtered calcium is passively reabsorbed in the proximal tubules. But, regulation of calcium reabsorption is in the distal nephrons. It is regulated by PTH by favouring calcium reabsorption in the loop of Henle and the distal convoluted tubule.

PTH stimulates the synthesis of 1-alpha hydroxylase in the proximal tubules, catalyses calcidiol conversion to calcitriol. PTH also decreases the activity of a 24-hydroxylase that inactivates calcitriol. Calcitriol is essential for intestinal absorption of calcium. The PTH-mediated action is crucial in maintaining normal calcium homeostasis and is deficient in vitamin D deficiency [42]. Calcitriol is essential for calcium absorption from the gut and thereby PTH enhances calcium absorption indirectly.

References

1. Sasou S, Nakamura S, Kurihara H. Suspensory ligament of berry: its relationship to recurrent laryngeal nerve and anatomic examination of 24 autopsies. Head Neck. 1998;20:695–8.
2. Henry BM, Sanna B, Graves MJ, Sanna S, Vikse J, Tomaszewska IM, Tubbs RS, Tomaszewski KA. The reliability of the tracheoesophageal groove and the ligament of berry as landmarks for identifying the recurrent laryngeal nerve: a cadaveric study and meta-analysis. Biomed Res Int. 2017;2017:4357591.

3. Pelizzo MR, Toniato A, Gemo G. Zuckerkandl's tuberculum: an arrow pointing to the recurrent laryngeal nerve (constant anatomical landmark). J Am Coll Surg. 1998;187:333–6.
4. James YE, Doleagbenou A, Kassegne I, Biramah BT, Keke K, Dosseh ED, Ayite AE, James K. Zuckerkandl's tubercle: incidence and relationship with the inferior laryngeal nerve. Morphology. 2014;98(323):171–5.
5. Berlin D, Lahey FH. The relationship of the recurrent laryngeal nerve to the inferior thyroid artery and the relationship of the superior to abduction paralysis. Surg Gynecol Obstet. 1929;49:102.
6. Polednak AP. Relationship of the recurrent laryngeal nerve to the inferior thyroid artery: a comparison of findings from two systematic reviews. Clin Anat. 2017;30(3):318–21. https://doi.org/10.1002/ca.22851.
7. Ling XY, Smoll NR. A systematic review of variations of the recurrent laryngeal nerve. Clin Anat. 2016;29(1):104–10.
8. Toniato A, Mazzarotto R, Piotto A, Bernante P, Pagetta C, Pelizzo MR. Identification of the nonrecurrent laryngeal nerve during thyroid surgery: 20-year experience. World J Surg. 2004;28(7):659–61.
9. Henry BM, Vikse J, Graves MJ, Sanna S, Sanna B, Tomaszewska IM, Tubbs RS, Tomaszewski KA. Extralaryngeal branching of the recurrent laryngeal nerve: a meta-analysis of 28,387 nerves. Langenbeck's Arch Surg. 2016;401(7):913–23.
10. Barczyński M, Stopa M, Konturek A, Nowak W. The overwhelming majority but not all motor fibers of the bifid recurrent laryngeal nerve are located in the anterior extralaryngeal branch. World J Surg. 2016;40(3):629–35.
11. Gurleyik E. Location of motor fibers within branches of the recurrent laryngeal nerve with extralaryngeal terminal bifurcation; Functional identification by intraoperative neuromonitoring. Surgery. 2015;158(5):1339–44.
12. Randolph GW, et al. Chapter 3. Surgical anatomy and monitoring of the recurrent laryngeal nerve. In: Surgery of the thyroid and parathyroid glands. 2nd ed. Elsevier; 2021. p. 306–16.
13. Cernea CR, Nishio S, Hojaji FC. Identification of the EBSLN in large goiters. Am J Otol. 1995;16:307–11.
14. Kierner AC, Aigner M, Burian M. The external branch of the superior laryngeal nerve: its topographical anatomy as related to surgery of the neck. Arch Otolaryngol Head Neck Surg. 1998;124:301–3.
15. Friedman M, Lo Savio P, Ibrahim H. Superior laryngeal nerve identification and preservation in thyroidectomy. Arch Otolaryngol Head Neck Surg. 2002;128:296–303.
16. Roy N, Smith ME, Dromey C, Redd J, Neff S, Grennan D. Exploring the phonatory effects of external superior laryngeal nerve paralysis: an in vivo model. Laryngoscope. 2009;119(4):816–26.
17. Wu BL, Sanders I, Mu L, Biller HF. The human communicating nerve. An extension of the external superior laryngeal nerve that innervates the vocal cord. Arch Otolaryngol Head Neck Surg. 1994;120(12):1321–8.
18. Sañudo JR, Maranillo E, Leon X, Mirapeix RM, Orus C, Quer M. An anatomical study of the anastomosis between the laryngeal nerves. Laryngoscope. 1999;109:983–7.
19. Naidu L, Ramsaroop L, Partab P, Satyapal KS. Galen's "anastomosis" revisited. Clin Anat. 2012;25(6):722–8. https://doi.org/10.1002/ca.22011.
20. Hodgson KJ, Lazarus JH, Wheeler MH. Duplex scan-derived thyroid blood flow in euthyroid and hyperthyroid patients. World J Surg. 1988;12(4):470.
21. Toni R, Della CC, Castorina S, Roti E, Ceda G, Valenti G. A meta-analysis of inferior thyroid artery variation in different human ethnic groups and their clinical implications. Ann Anat. 2005;187:371–85.
22. Johansson K, Ander S, Lennquist S, Smeds S. Human parathyroid blood supply determined by laser-Doppler flowmetry. World J Surg. 1994;18(3):417–20.
23. Nobori M, Saiki S, Tanaka N, Harihara Y, Shindo S, Fujimoto Y. Blood supply of the parathyroid gland from the superior thyroid artery. Surgery. 1994;115(4):417–23.

24. Hollinshead WH. Anatomy for surgeons, vol. 1. 3rd ed. Philadelphia: Lippincott Williams and Wilkins; 1982.
25. Arrangoiz R, Cordera F, Caba D, Muñoz M, Moreno E, de León EL. Comprehensive review of thyroid embryology, anatomy, histology, and physiology for surgeons. International Journal of Otolaryngy. 2018;7:160–88.
26. Mitevska E, Gerasimovska Z, Milenkova L, Kostovska N. Histological structure of the thyroid gland in apolipoprotein E deficient female mice after levothyroxine application. Pril (Makedon Akad Nauk Umet Odd Med Nauki). 2014;35(3):135–40.
27. Shoyele O, Bacus B, Haddad L, Li Y, Shidham V. Lymphoproliferative process with reactive follicular cells in thyroid fine-needle aspiration: a few simple but important diagnostic pearls. Cytojournal. 2019;16:20.
28. Shah JP. Thyroid carcinoma: epidemiology, histology, and diagnosis. Clin Adv Hematol Oncol. 2015;13(4 Suppl 4):3–6.
29. Rousset B, Dupuy C, Miot F, et al. Chapter 2. Thyroid hormone synthesis and secretion. In: Feingold KR, Anawalt B, Boyce A, et al., editors. Endotext. South Dartmouth, MA: MDText.com, Inc.; 2000. https://www.ncbi.nlm.nih.gov/books/NBK285550.
30. Feingold KR, Anawalt B, Boyce A, et al., editors. Endotext. South Dartmouth, MA: MDText.com, Inc.; 2000. https://www.ncbi.nlm.nih.gov/books/NBK285550
31. Kopp P, Pesce L, Solis JC. Pendred syndrome and iodide transport in the thyroid. Trend Endocrinol Metab. 2008;19:260–8.
32. Massart C, Hoste C, Virion A, Ruf J, Dumont JE, Van Sande J. Cell biology of H(2)O(2) generation in the thyroid: investigation of the control of dual oxidases (DUOX) activity in intact ex vivo thyroid tissue and cell lines. Mol Cell Endocrinol. 2011;343(1–2):32–44.
33. Collip JB. The extraction of a parathyroid hormone will prevent or control parathyroid tetany and which regulates the level of blood calcium. J Biol Chem. 1925;63:395–438.
34. Rasmussen H, Craig LC. Purification of parathormone by use of countercurrent distribution. J Am Chem Soc. 1959;81:5003.
35. Munger BL, Roth SI. The cytology of the normal parathyroid glands of man and Virginia deer; a light and electron microscopic study with morphologic evidence of secretory activity. J Cell Biol. 1963;16:379–400.
36. Christie AC. The parathyroid oxyphil cells. J Clin Pathol. 1967;20(4):591–602.
37. Ritter CS, Haughey BH, Miller B, Brown AJ. Differential gene expression by oxyphil and chief cells of human parathyroid glands. J Clin Endocrinol Metab. 2012;97(8):E1499–505. https://doi.org/10.1210/jc.2011-3366. Epub 2012 May 14.
38. Naveh-Many T, Silver J, Kronenberg HM. Parathyroid hormone molecular biology. In: Bilezikian JP, Martin TJ, Clemens TL, Rosen CJ, editors. Principles of bone biology, vol. 1. 4th ed. San Diego, CA: Elsevier; 2019. p. 575.
39. Centeno PP, Herberger A, Mun HC, Tu C, Nemeth EF, Chang W, Conigrave AD, Ward DT. Phosphate acts directly on the calcium-sensing receptor to stimulate parathyroid hormone secretion. Nat Commun. 2019;10(1):4693. https://doi.org/10.1038/s41467-019-12399-9.
40. Canaff L, Hendy GN. Human calcium-sensing receptor gene. Vitamin D response elements in promoters P1 and P2 confer transcriptional responsiveness to 1,25-dihydroxyvitamin D. J Biol Chem. 2002;277(33):30337–50. https://doi.org/10.1074/jbc.M201804200. Epub 2002 May 29.
41. Martin A, David V, Quarles LD. Regulation and function of the FGF23/klotho endocrine pathways. Physiol Rev. 2012;92(1):131–55. https://doi.org/10.1152/physrev.00002.2011.
42. Silva BC, Bilezikian JP. Parathyroid hormone: anabolic and catabolic actions on the skeleton. Curr Opin Pharmacol. 2015;22:41–50. https://doi.org/10.1016/j.coph.2015.03.005.

5 Pre-operative Counselling

C. Gopalakrishnan Nair, Riju Ramachandran, and Pradeep Jacob

The majority of patients reporting for thyroidectomy are asymptomatic and the operation necessitates the need for lifelong thyroxine supplementation exposing them to many potential complications with lasting effects. It is absolutely necessary that every patient is educated appropriately for ideal postoperative care.

The majority of patients are operated on under General Anaesthesia with endotracheal intubation. Thyroidectomy is a procedure of removing an essential structure and results in permanent changes. These patients are at risk of complications that have life-long effects. So proper counselling is absolutely essential. Counselling is always done by one of the senior members of the surgical team and close relative/ relatives of the patient are also invited to accompany the patient.

Counselling is a continuous procedure that starts when thyroidectomy is planned as the line of treatment. The reasons to opt for this surgical option are explained in detail. A very common query from the patient at this point is whether the procedure is to be done as an emergency. The suggestion of thyroidectomy is often an unexpected option and the patient may need time to make an informed decision. The surgeons' opinion is almost always individualised and based on the case scenario. But the authors feel that patients and relatives should be given adequate time to make the final decision.

The gross anatomy and an outline of the function of thyroid hormone are explained avoiding all scientific terms. The outline of the procedure is given in simple words making it clear that the procedure aims to remove the gland completely or partially. Often, many patients are perplexed as to the need for removing an entire gland when a simple removal of the nodule should have sufficed.

C. G. Nair (✉)
Professor of Surgery, Endocrine Surgery Division, Amrita Institute of Medical Sciences and Research Centre, Kochi, Kerala, India

R. Ramachandran · P. Jacob
Department of Surgery, AIMS, Kochi, Kochi, Kerala, India

C. G. Nair, S. J. Abraham (eds.), *Surgical Management of Thyroid and Parathyroid Diseases*, https://doi.org/10.1007/978-981-97-3774-1_5

Patients who are opting for diagnostic hemithyroidectomy shall be adequately informed of the possibility of a second surgery—a completion thyroidectomy. The benefits of hemithyroidectomy far outweigh the hazards of the second surgery in many aspects. The surgeon should assure the patient that there shall be no increase in the complication rate during the excision of the thyroid gland, even if it is done as a staged procedure.

The definite sequel of the open procedure is a scar and the surgeon should not assure the patient of cosmesis since the fate of the scar is very unpredictable. The anterior neck is mostly uncovered in the usual code of dressing and patients are nervous of consenting to procedures on the region. Patients who are very concerned about scars may be channelled to remote access procedures. They should be informed of selection criteria for such procedures and additional specific complications related to those procedures.

Hormone supplementation is essential following total thyroidectomy and good compliance is expected. Some patients may also require hormone supplementation following hemithyroidectomy. It is not uncommon for the layperson to be ignorant of hormones and their relevance in normal hemopoiesis. The patient has to be educated regarding the broad outline of functions of thyroid hormone and its relevance to ensure compliance with hormone supplementation. Many patients express a sceptical view on the long-term dependence on drugs. They are assured that the tablets contain synthetic analogue of naturally occurring thyroxine.

Thyroidectomy is a major operation and approximately 1% may have major immediate life-threatening complications, reactionary bleeding and haematoma. The chances of complications like hypocalcaemia and laryngeal nerve palsy are seen in 2% of patients. Awareness of these complications is a deterring factor to many patients. The counsellor has to present all information but should not undermine the patient's confidence.

There are few other less severe but very disturbing complications. Thyroidectomy is always performed in a supine position with neck extension. Overstretching of the cervical spine may cause neck pain and cervical radiculopathy.

Transverse cervical nerve (cutaneous nerve) courses through the subcutaneous plane deep to the platysma and supplies the anterior neck. The nerve is at risk while the flap is dissected and can cause paraesthesia or anaesthesia of the region.

Counsellors should be cautious when discussing these deterring issues since overzealous emphasis may attract a negative decision. Thyroidectomy is considered as treatment with curative intent with a near 100% success rate in conditions like nodular goitre, hyperthyroidism and differentiated thyroid carcinoma. A high cure rate with a low rate of postoperative complications shall be highlighted to win over the patient's indecisiveness.

Counselling is a continuous process that starts when the decision of thyroidectomy is made. Most of the patients and relatives are overwhelmed by the simple suggestion of operation and are not in a mindset to receive the counsellor's words. So printed brochures in simple language avoiding scientific terms help provide preliminary information. We found that the second session of counselling was more helpful in achieving the patient's confidence.

Thyroidectomy: Steps of Procedure

6

C. Gopalakrishnan Nair, Riju Ramachandran,
and Pradeep Jacob

6.1 Introduction

Thyroidectomy is a clean surgical procedure and preoperative antibiotic administration is not required. All patients are instructed to take a bath with medicated soap and clipping of hair of male patients done on the day of surgery.

Thyroidectomy is a very delicate surgical procedure and requires patience and dedication. Laryngeal nerves and parathyroid glands require careful handling. Soft-tissue dissection should be precise and should not be excessive since the resulting fibrosis causes a lasting tightening sensation. Excessive stretching and division of strap muscles occasionally cause temporary voice changes. The intensity of diathermy should be reduced when handling skin flaps since deeper burns may cause marks on the skin.

Steps:

1. The incision is marked in the normal sitting position with a permanent marker pen before the patient is moved to the operation room. The incision is planned 1.5 cm above the suprasternal notch approximately 6–8 cm in length, passing equidistant to each side in a curvilinear fashion. Adequate care is taken to have equal length on both sides. The scar moves down to the chest wall if a low incision is made in large volume goitres (Fig. 6.1a–c).
2. Anaesthesia—General anaesthesia administered through an oral endotracheal tube is preferred. Infiltration of local anaesthetic agents to block cervical plexus is an option but generally requires adequate sedation. Mobilisation of the thyroid gland from the trachea is disturbing to many patients when thyroidectomy is performed under the cervical block (Fig. 6.2).

C. G. Nair (✉)
Professor of Surgery, Endocrine Surgery Division, Amrita Institute of Medical Sciences and Research Centre, Kochi, Kerala, India

R. Ramachandran · P. Jacob
Department of Surgery, AIMS, Kochi, Kochi, Kerala, India

C. G. Nair, S. J. Abraham (eds.), *Surgical Management of Thyroid and Parathyroid Diseases*, https://doi.org/10.1007/978-981-97-3774-1_6

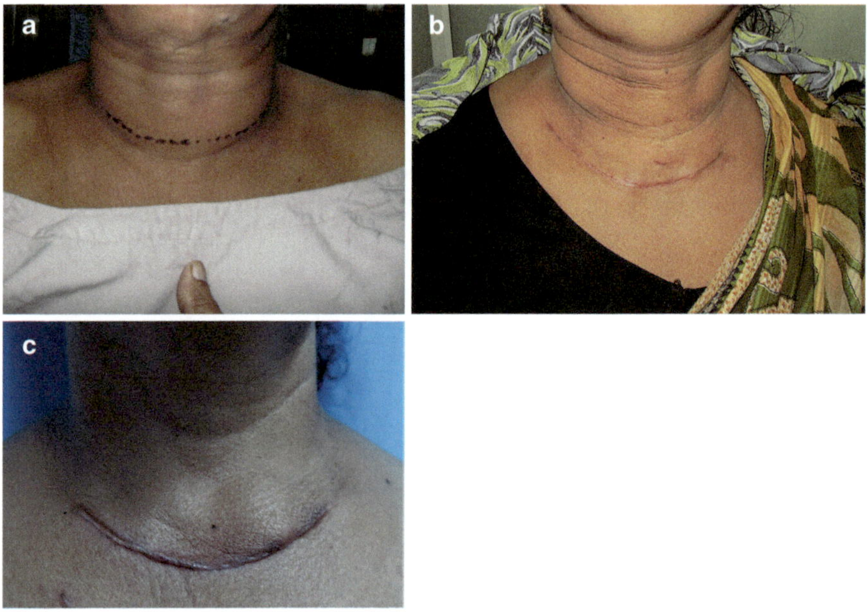

Fig. 6.1 (**a**) Planning incision P1.JPG. (**b**) Bad untidy scar. (**c**) Bad scar P1 b

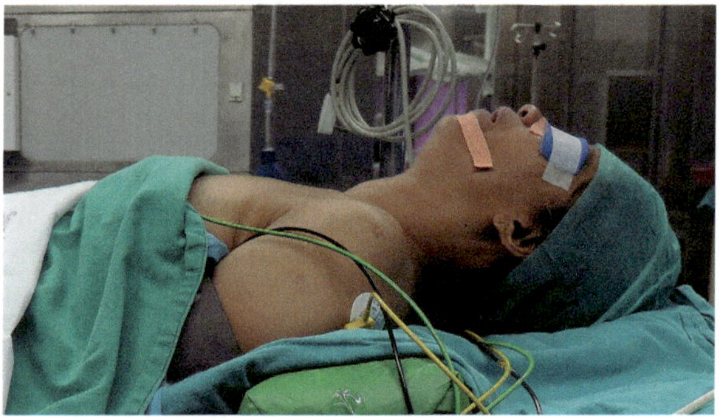

Fig. 6.2 General anesthesia with endotracheal intubation was completed

3. Positioning—The patient is positioned supine with shoulder roll or gel pad at the level of the acromion process (Fig. 6.3a). Positioning is done with care to protect the cervical spine since the patient is under muscle relaxant. The head is to be steadied with a ring to prevent rolling. It is advisable to avoid overzealous extension especially in the person having cervical spondylosis. The upper limbs are kept close to the body and are tucked safely on either side. The neck is further exposed by gently drawing the upper limbs down while tucking on the side (Fig. 6.3b).

   There are few markedly obese patients with short neck which limits the exposure of the anterior neck. Overzealous attempts to extend the neck should be avoided since it may result in postoperative neck pain or even cervical radic-

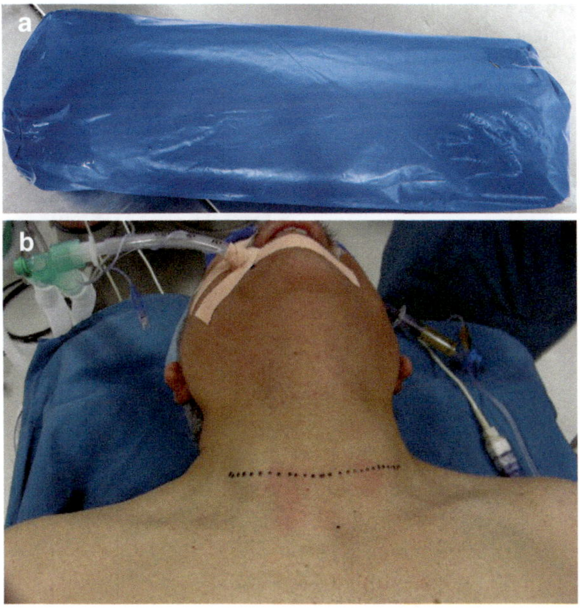

Fig. 6.3 (**a**) Shoulder pillow. (**b**) Position; the patient positioned for thyroidectomy

ulopathy. In obese females with bulky breasts gentle traction exerted on the breasts and anchored to the anterior abdominal wall with adhesive tapes opens the neck sufficiently

4. Painting and draping—Before painting the surgical site, ensure proper positions of ECG leads and other points of contact of patient monitoring systems. Ten percent Povidone-iodine solution contains 10 mg of iodine in 1 mL and was considered to increase the iodine load of the body by absorption through the skin [1]. Chlorhexidine gluconate solution is another alternative for skin preparation. Skin preparation should reach beyond the chin and to the anterior chest wall up to the fourth rib and well on to the sides of the neck. Drapes cover the head and expose the anterior aspect of the neck (Fig. 6.3c).

   The patient is properly connected to energy sources and the intensity of the diathermy equipment suction apparatus is adjusted to a suitable level (Fig. 6.4).
5. The operating team is ideally formed by the main surgeon with two fellows and a scrub nurse. The main surgeon and one colleague stand on the right side; the other colleague and scrub nurse remain on the left side. It is preferable to keep a Mayo trolley behind draping towards the abdomen of the patient for spreading the necessary instruments (Fig. 6.5a).
6. Instruments commonly used include (Fig. 6.5b):
   (a) Bard-Parker handle with #15 blade
   (b) Pair of Joseph skin hook
   (c) Pair of Allis Tissue holding forceps (6″)
   (d) Pair of Babcock's forceps (159 cm)
   (e) Langenbeck retractor (4.1 cm × 1.27 cm) 4 numbers

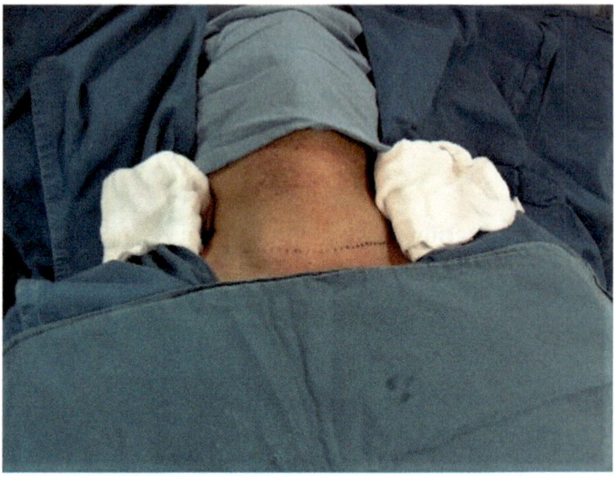

Fig. 6.4 Draping completed

(f) Curved mosquito forceps—6
(g) Kelly haemostatic forceps (7″)—3
(h) Right angle forceps—2
(i) DeBakey thumb forceps (8″)—2
(j) Pair of Adson forceps
(k) Haemostatic clips (small and medium) with applicators
(l) Mayo needle holder (6″)
(m) Metzenbaum curved scissors—1
(n) Suture cutting scissors—1
(o) Energy sources for haemostasis: Electrosurgical equipment inducing monopolar and bipolar thermal coagulation is adequate for routine surgery. Monopolar device is to be avoided near any vital structures since lateral spread is more than 10 mm. Bipolar devises can seal of vessels up to 7 mm diameter and lateral spread of temperature is approximately 4 mm.
(p) Harmonic scalpel and Ligasure instruments have less temperature at the instrument tips and lateral spread is approximately 2.5 mm. These devices are useful when laryngeal nerves are close to the gland.

7. Incision—The first assistant stretches the skin on the chest side while the surgeon holds the skin steady on the other side. The knife should be held perpendicular to the skin so that an oblique skin cut is avoided. Further deepening of the incision may be done using the cutting mode of diathermy to divide the subcutaneous tissue and platysma keeping the intensity low to avoid thermal injury of the skin. Skin edge bleeding is generally minimal but can be troublesome when a patient has retro-sternal extension compressing the venous flow (Fig. 6.6a–c).
8. Development of skin flaps—An avascular plane is exposed with traction given on the skin hooks held in the left hand of the first assistant and gentle pressure exerted on the raw surface with the right hand. The skin flaps are made in a subplatysmal plane up to the thyroid notch in the cephalic direction. The lower flap is raised to expose the Space of Burns. Superficial veins are distended and

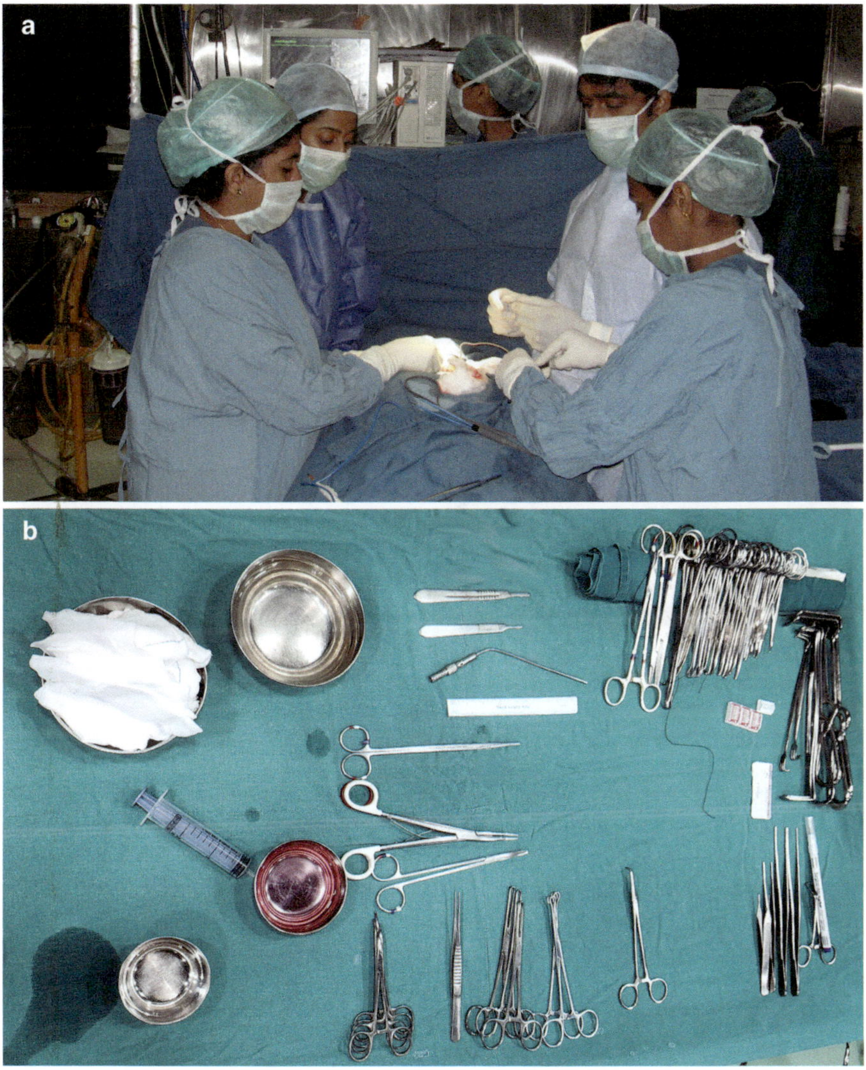

Fig. 6.5 The operating team

tortuous in patients with mediastinal extension hence adequate care should be given not to injure them. The flaps are held with stay sutures taken through subcutaneous tissue close to the edge anchored to drapes. A self-retaining retractor like Joll thyroid retractor may be used instead of stay sutures. (Fig. 6.7a–e).

9. Division of investing layer of deep fascia—Two retractors are placed to expose the midline one at the level of the thyroid cartilage and one at the sternoclavicular joint. The first assistant may hold them steady while the midline is divided. The division is done craniocaudal in the midline through an avascular plane

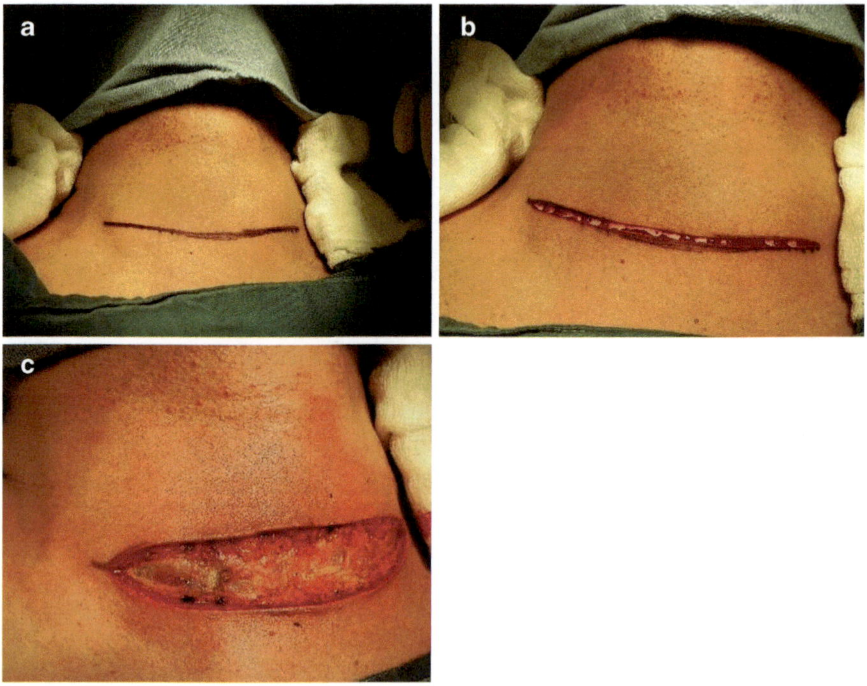

Fig. 6.6 Incision and division of platysma

between the strap muscles on either side. But actual midline may be shifted to one side in patients with large volume goitre with dissimilar enlargement. The avascular plane can be reached from below or from the thyroid notch above. Adequate care is given not to injure the anterior jugular veins and communicating vein in the Burns Space (Fig. 6.8a–c).

10. The investing layer and strap muscles are steadied with Allis tissue, holding forceps and gentle traction will expose the surface of the thyroid gland. (Mobilisation of the thyroid is initiated on one side, actually, the choice is based on the surgeon's preference. The authors prefer to start with the right lobe first.) The right lobe is mobilised by separating the strap muscles from the anterior aspect. The second assistant standing on the side of the surgeon steadies the tissue holding forceps and the first assistant on the other side exerts gentle traction on the lobe to the left side. Using sharp dissection with bipolar forceps the strap muscles are separated from the lobe. This plane is always avascular but bleeding may occur from surface veins by overzealous traction or improper usage of diathermy. The Allis forceps are removed on reaching the lateral aspect and the Langenbeck retractor is introduced. Gentle traction exerted on the retractor exposes the lateral surface (Fig. 6.9a, b).
11. Strap muscles are generally separable from the gland with an avascular plane. Thyroid cancers infiltrate the strap muscles (commonly the sternothyroid) are found adherent to the gland. Sternothyroid muscle can be excised in full length

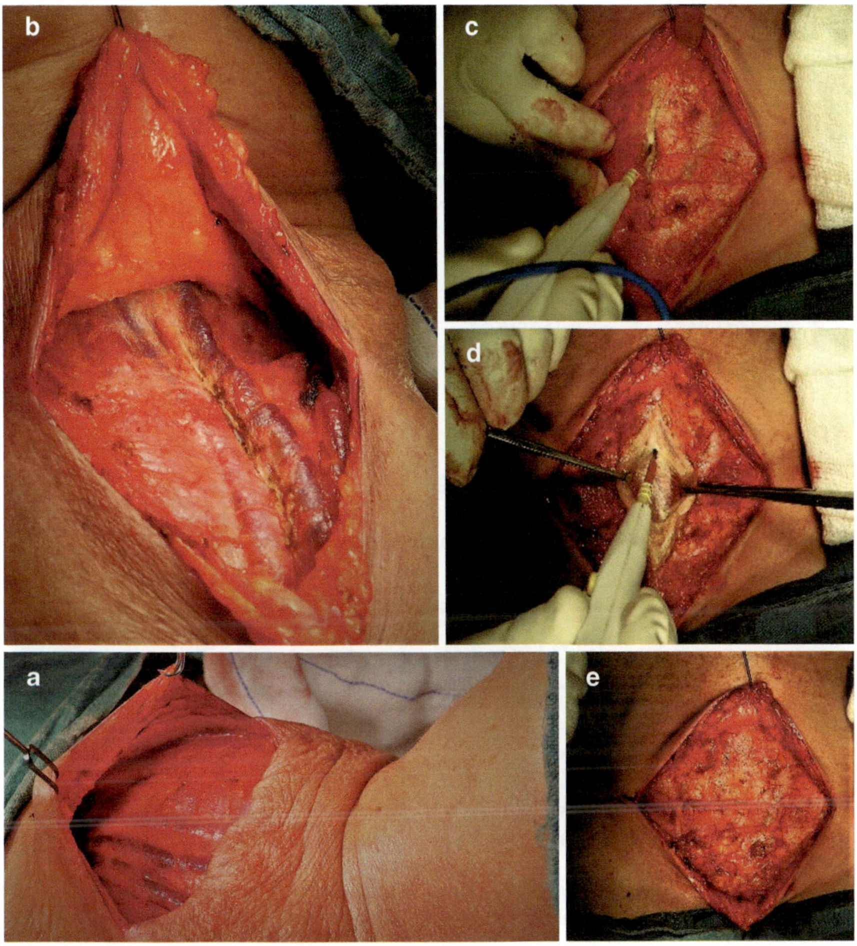

Fig. 6.7 (**a**) Upper flap. (**b**) Anchoring the flaps for exposure

along with the thyroid. Sternothyroid and thyrohyoid are removed along with the thyroid gland if malignant infiltration is suspected. The second assistant holds the muscle steady while division is done using bipolar diathermy. Bleeding vessels are carefully controlled with diathermy.

In large volume goitres, the lateral mobilisation may require partial or complete division of strap muscle. If the division is necessary the ansa cervicalis is preserved at the lateral border of the sternothyroid muscle.

12. The lobe of the thyroid is freed from the strap muscles by sharp dissection. The first assistant from the opposite side holds the lobe medially either with fingers or a lightweight Babcock tissue holding forceps. These manoeuvres expose the structures on the lateral aspect of the lobe. Middle thyroid veins are seen in 30% of patients and are clipped, or burned with energy sources close to the thyroid. Occasionally the third vein of Kocher is observed closer to the lower pole and

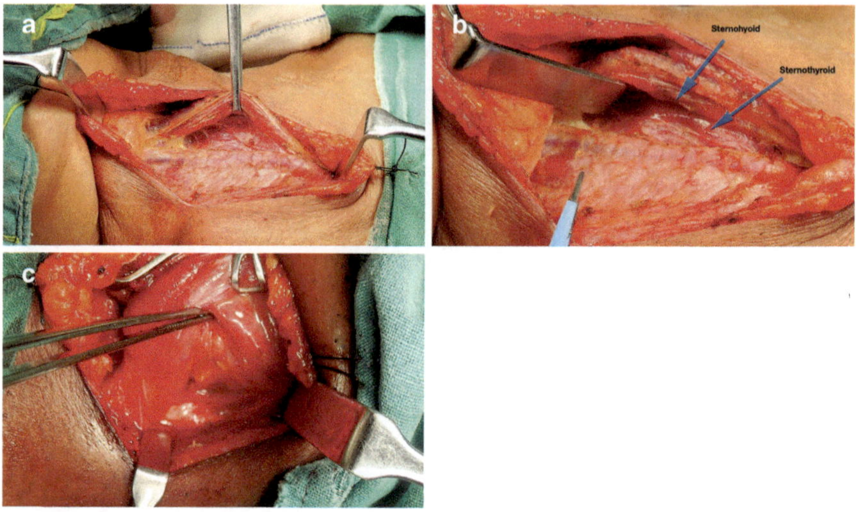

Fig. 6.8 Ant jug vein and incising the investing layer cervical fascia in midline

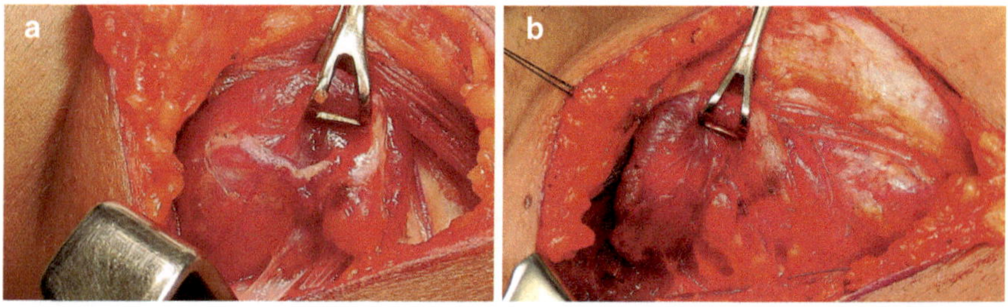

Fig. 6.9 Strap muscles. (**a**) Opening the fascia and retracting strap muscle in the midline. (**b**) Sternothyroid and sternohyoid muscles. Lateral dissection of strap muscle in adherent gland

another vein is seen closer to the superior pole. The upper pole of the thyroid is mobilised on the lateral aspect from the carotid sheath. Careful dissection is mandatory since this is a common site of malignant infiltration in advanced thyroid cancers. Encasement of the carotid artery by malignant infiltration occurs at this site. The lateral dissection is carried out to reach the pre-vertebral fascia taking care not to injure the sympathetic chain. The superior thyroid artery is well-taken care of only after the lateral aspect is mobilised (Fig. 6.10a–c).

13. Exposure of superior pole—Sterno-thyroid closely hugs the superior pole of thyroid and may require the division to expose it. Two well-placed Langenbeck retractors (one placed laterally retracting strap muscles and sternomastoid muscle; another placed cephalopod direction holding the sterno-thyroid insertion) help to expose the superior pole. The lateral retractor is applied cautiously to avoid traction on the carotid sheath. A lightweight Babcock forceps are care-

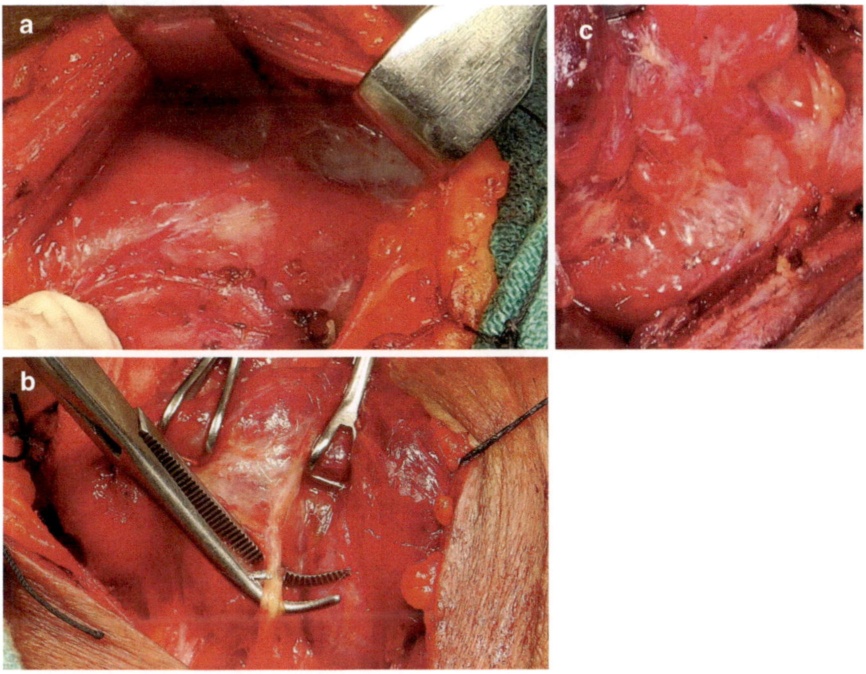

Fig. 6.10 Middle thyroid vein

fully used to hold the gland pulling the pole outward exposes the cricothyroid space.

The nodules from the superior pole grow deep to SCM and the vessels stretch on the surface of it. The nodule is delivered gently by retracting the strap muscles laterally (Fig. 6.11a–c).

14. The space between the superior pole and cricothyroid space is known as cricothyroid space which is usually avascular. The superior pole is dissected free and external division of the superior laryngeal nerve (EBSLN) is identified. Langenbeck retractor placed to retract the SCM is steadied by the assistant on the left side of the surgeon while a second retractor is placed to retract the sternothyroid. The space is usually avascular but the division of the superior thyroid artery to pyramidal lobe may course through the space. The EBSLN crosses the artery at a variable level and is seen descending parallel to the artery. The soft tissue is better dissected free before energy souse is used to avoid thermal damage to the nerve. After the cricothyroid space is defined and EBSLN is located the STA is hooked using right-angle forceps and burned or clipped as the preference of the surgeon. When the upper pole extends cephaloid the stump of the STA is held by DeBakey and freed from the thyroid. The vein which accompanies the artery is now exposed and treated in a similar fashion. The superior pole is dissected off the remaining soft tissue up to the level of isthmus medially. Adequate care is given on the lateral aspect since RLN may have a sinuous course and close to the thyroid (Fig. 6.12a–d).

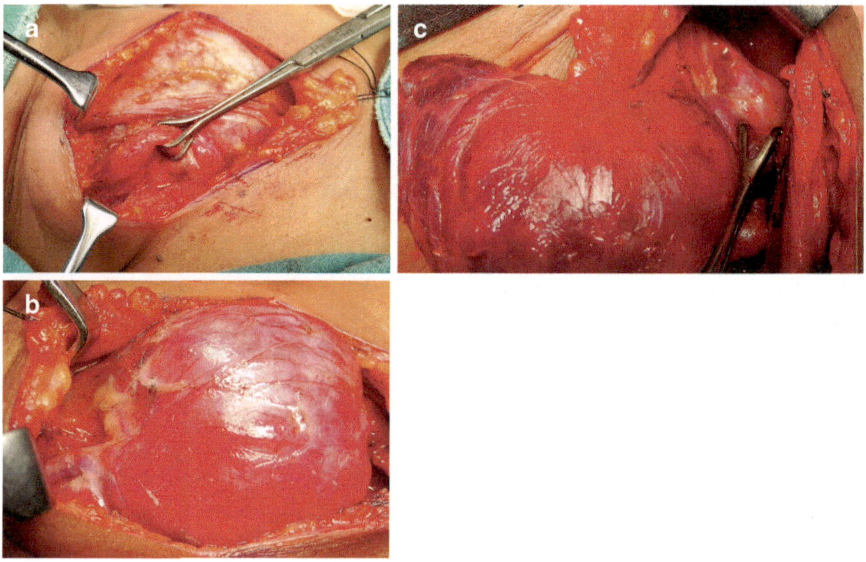

Fig. 6.11 Superior pole dissection

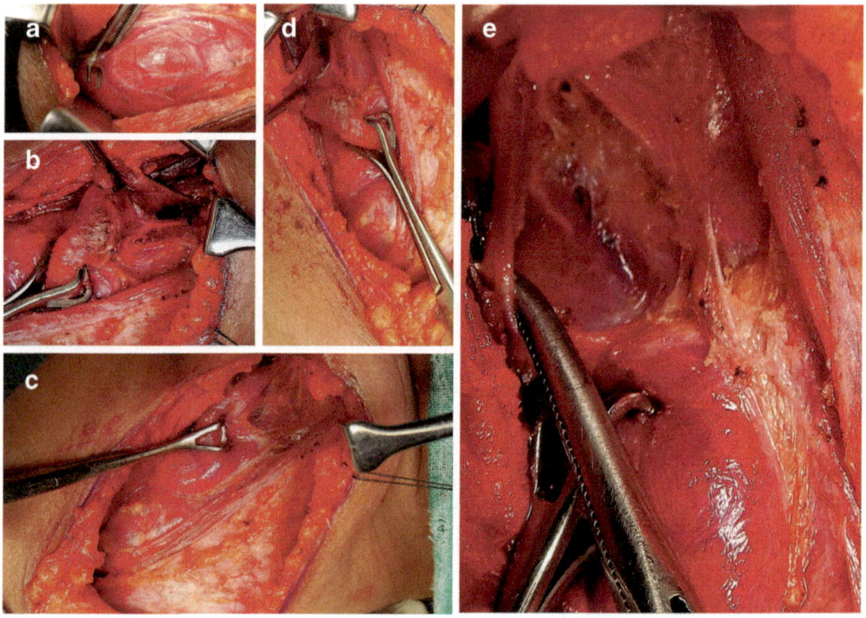

Fig. 6.12 (**a**) Superior pedicle. (**b–d**) Sup. Thyroid artery and EBSLN in the cricothyroid space. (**e**) Superior thyroid artery ligation. Nerve crossing the cricothyroid space

15. The dissection is continued on the lateral aspect of the lobe to separate it from the strap muscle. The lobe is gently held medially by the assistant on the opposite side. A Langenbeck retractor is placed laterally retracting the strap muscles and SCM exposing the peri-thyroidal soft tissue. The middle thyroid vein (if not divided earlier) and the third veins of Kocher are visible now and divided (Fig. 6.13).
16. The pre-tracheal fascia is a thin loose layer covering the lobe. This fascia is held with a DeBakey forceps and is stripped of the thyroid gland using bipolar forceps. The energy source has to be used with caution towards the posterior aspect since the RLN and posterior anastomotic plexus of arteries may be encountered. Rarely the recurrent laryngeal nerve may course more anteriorly especially in large volume goitres (Fig. 6.14a–c).
17. The terminal divisions of the Inferior Thyroid Artery (ITA) are seen entering the gland on the lateral aspect. These vessels are cautiously secured and divided.

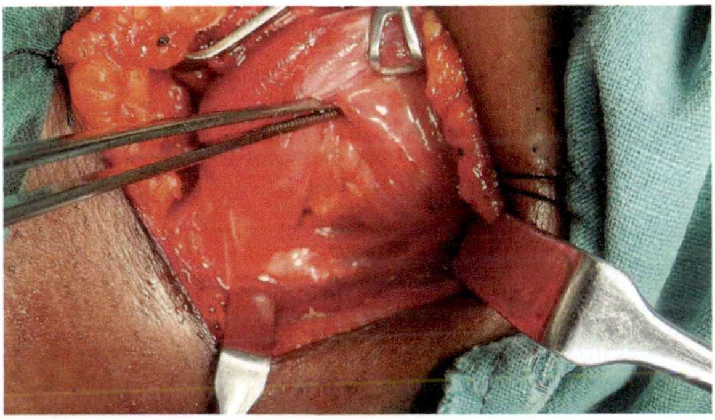

Fig. 6.13 Lateral lobe mobilisation

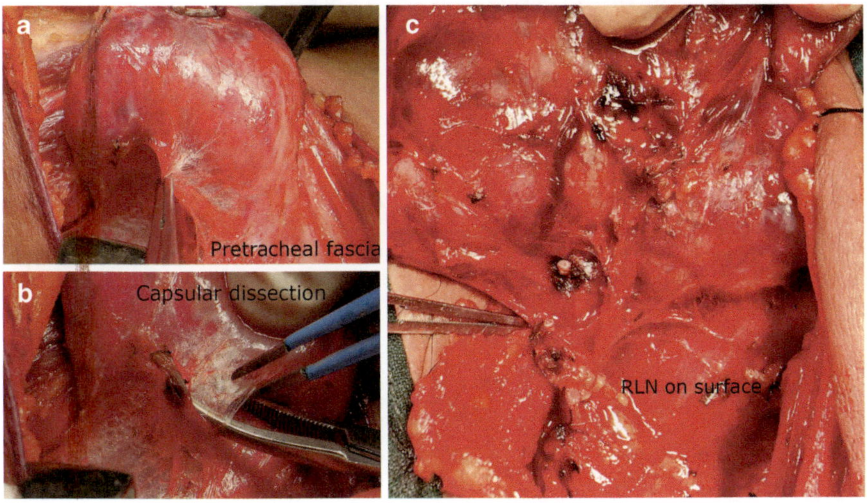

Fig. 6.14 Capsular dissection

(Slipped end of arterial branches bleeds profusely and retracts close to the RLN. Indiscriminate use of haemostat is dangerous in this situation.)

The first assistant maintains medial retraction of the lobe while the second assistant holds the retractor laterally exposing the lateral lobe. The bleeding vessel is controlled by applying pressure using a wet gauze for 2–3 min. The light is adjusted to focus the area and gauze is released slowly and the pulsating end is seen. The cut end of the vessel is held with DeBakey forceps and haemostatic clip is applied.

Towards the superior pole, the superior parathyroid glands are seen in close approximation to the posterior border gland. The parathyroid artery may be coursing in relation posterior border of the lobe. The energy sources should be used carefully to protect the vessel (Fig. 6.15a–c).

18. Tubercle of Zuckerkandl (TZ) is a good landmark when identifiable and the RLN is found posterior, inferior, or even lateral to the tubercle. TZ is inconspicuous in many thyroids but found significantly enlarged in a few nodular goitres. Inferior parathyroid also may have variable relation to the tubercle as found above or lateral to the tubercle (Refer to pictures in Anatomy).

    TZ is not always visible and is not a constant landmark of RLN. False capsule of the thyroid is further stripped down towards the trachea-oesophageal grove where the recurrent laryngeal nerve is exposed. But the course of RLN is not constant and a very oblique course towards the point of entry to the larynx is not uncommon on the right side (Fig. 6.16a–c).
19. Right recurrent laryngeal nerve is not constantly found related to the trachea-oesophageal grove and variations in course and relationships are more frequently encountered on the right side. The nerve is occasionally found to course obliquely to the point of entry to the larynx. The false capsule is stripped down

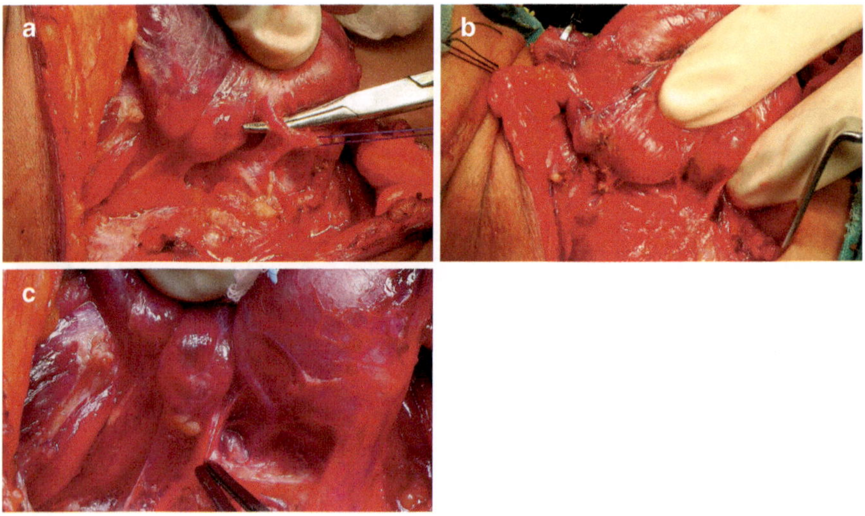

Fig. 6.15 ITA ligation

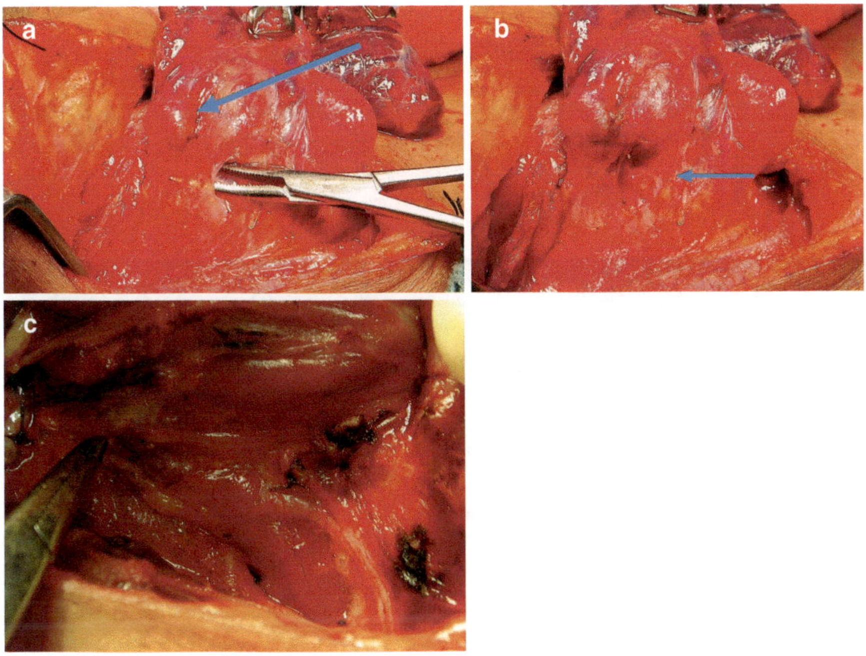

Fig. 6.16 RLN and tubercle of Zuckerkandl

cautiously to expose the lower border of the thyroid lobe. This manoeuvre exposes the superior parathyroid and RLN near the point of entry.

A tonsil forceps is introduced above the line of nerve gently lifting the tubercle. The soft tissue adhesions are mostly avascular and released with bipolar diathermy taking care of the nerve. Turning the intensity of the energy source low and using wet saline gauze to cover the nerve help to protect it (Fig. 6.17a–d).

20. The left RLN is usually encountered in the trachea-oesophageal grove and is mostly seen on stripping the fascia down. But there is a higher chance of the nerve coursing on the surface of the lobe in large volume goitres. The energy sources should be used cautiously to safeguard the RLN when the capsule is stripped of the lobe (Fig. 6.18a–c).
21. After the RLN is exposed close to the thyroid gland, further dissection of the proximal part is not necessary if central compartment dissection is not planned. Mobilisation of the lower pole of the thyroid shall commence now. The dissection of the lower pole to separate the gland from the trachea includes identification and preservation of the inferior parathyroid gland with its blood supply and division of inferior thyroid veins. The Langenbeck retractor is placed close to the lower third of the sternocleidomastoid and the third assistant shall move to the right side of the main surgeon. The first assistant holds the lobe exerting mild traction towards the medial and cephaloid direction. The inferior thyroid veins or plexus of veins will be exposed now.

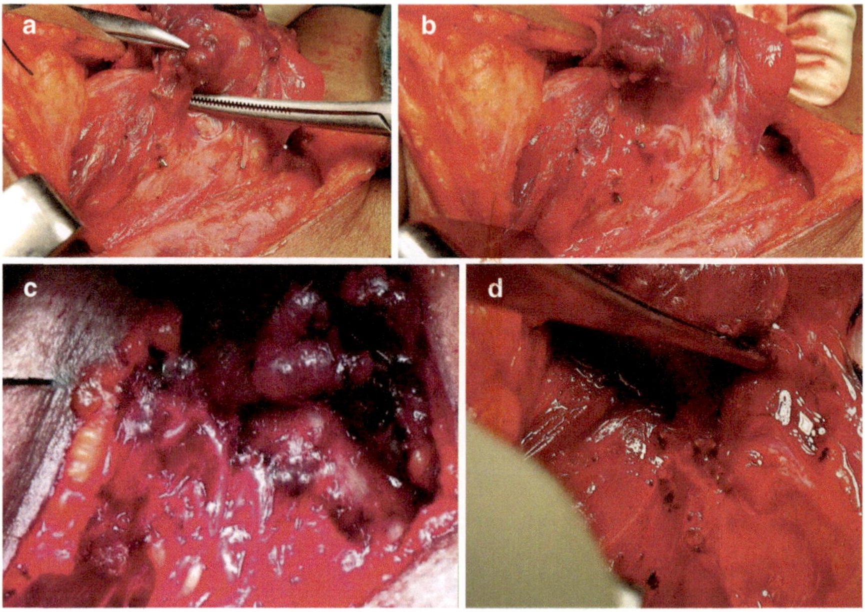

Fig. 6.17 RLN dissection continued

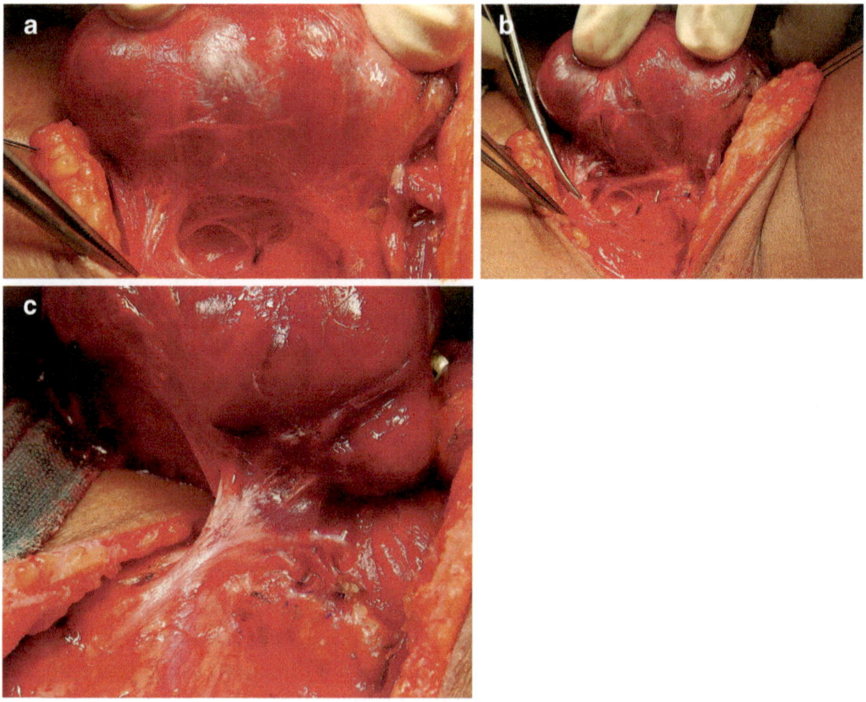

Fig. 6.18 (**a**) Left RLN dissection. (**b**, **c**) Left RLN

The course of recurrent laryngeal nerve is noted to avoid thermal damage of the nerve. Location of the inferior parathyroid gland is variable and so is looked for on the surface of the gland, paratracheal grove and anterior aspect of trachea approximately 1 cm vicinity form the lower pole. The parathyroid appears as a tiny piece of chocolate embedded in butter. When the parathyroid is not clearly identified dissection is kept close to the thyroid gland. It is equally important to preserve the vascular pedicle of the parathyroid which may arise from the trunk or from one of the divisions of ITA.

Inferior thyroid veins are secured by either bipolar diathermy or haemostatic clips. The soft tissue is divided with bipolar diathermy exposing the trachea and the lobe is further separated from the trachea. This manoeuvre is facilitated by holding the lobe steady with traction exerted towards the medial and cephaloid directions. The dissection is performed close to the lower border of the lobe to safeguard RLN and parathyroid vessels. The lobe and isthmus are separated from the trachea taking care of additional blood supply of thyroid from tracheal vessels. These vessels assume considerable significance in hyperthyroidism (Fig. 6.19).

22. Further dissection of the nerve towards the terminal portion is technically demanding especially on the right side. Good exposure and adequate lighting are very essential. The first assistant holds the lobe medially with a steady hand while the second assistant holds the retractor laterally.

    The nerve may be sinuous and close to the entrance to the larynx. Further pre-laryngeal branching may add to the complexity of the situation. It is of paramount importance to maintain perfect haemostasis since an inadequately controlled bleeder will retract close to the nerve.

23. Superior parathyroid gland is relatively constant in its location close to the posterior border of the upper pole of the thyroid. The parathyroid has different relations with the terminal portion of the RLN and occasionally covers it partially.

    Langenbeck retractor is placed to retract the strap muscles and sternocleidomastoid muscles laterally. The retractor is held by the third assistant on the left

Fig. 6.19 Dissection of RLN at the entry to the larynx

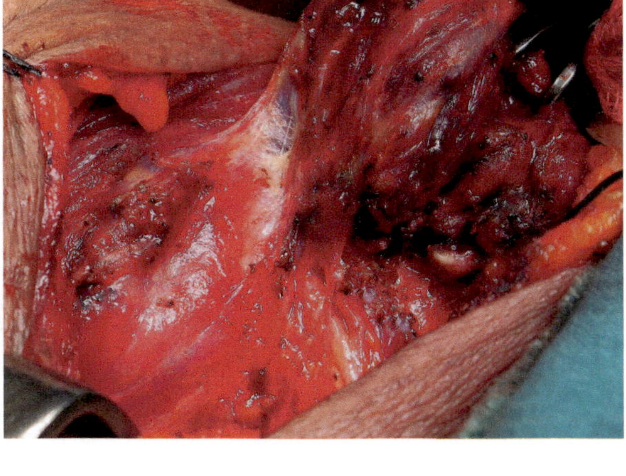

side of the operating surgeon. He/she has to be standing on the side to facilitate the free movement of the main surgeon.

Tip of tonsil forceps is gently negotiated in the line of nerve but superficial to it. The superior pole of the lobe is held with lightweight Babcock forceps to exert a mild taction. The soft tissue is lifted carefully to avoid excessive traction which may tear it. Bipolar diathermy using a microtip in low intensity is a valuable aid in this manoeuvre. The trunk of RLN or the anterior division coursing close to the posterior border of the thyroid or through the ligament of Berry mess up further dissection.

Occasionally a significant amount of thyroid tissue is present in the ligament of Berry. It is advisable to leave the posterior capsule or residual tissue in the ligament of Berry if closer dissection is suspected to damage the parathyroid blood supply or RLN. Cold saline is sprayed to the area will reduce the lateral thermal spread when energy sources are applied close to RLN and parathyroid glands.

Leaving behind residual tissue is not always advisable in conditions like medullary thyroid carcinoma. Sharp dissection using a number 16 blade can be attempted with precision and care to avoid bleeding. Judicious use of bipolar diathermy with micro tips at low intensity is recommended (Fig. 6.20a–f).

Inferior parathyroid glands were identified and preserved during the early phase of mobilisation (Fig. 6.21a, b).

24. Thyro-thymic rests are seen in approximately 10% of patients and assume great significance in patients with Graves' disease and thyroid cancers. The rests appear as tongue-like extensions or as tiny nodule-like lymph nodes below the lower pole. Occasionally nodules may arise from the rests extending to the superior mediastinum (Fig. 6.22).
25. The pre-tracheal fascia is open at the lower aspect and the goitre may extend to the superior mediastinum. Rarely nodules from the posterior aspect of the lobe can extend to the posterior mediastinum and grossly alter the course of RLN. Thyro-thymic rests can be independent islets of thyroid tissue and act as a

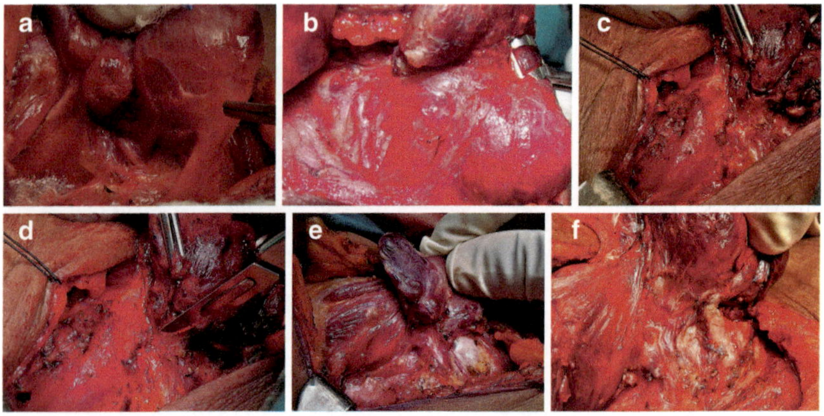

Fig. 6.20 Dissection of Parathyroid and RLN

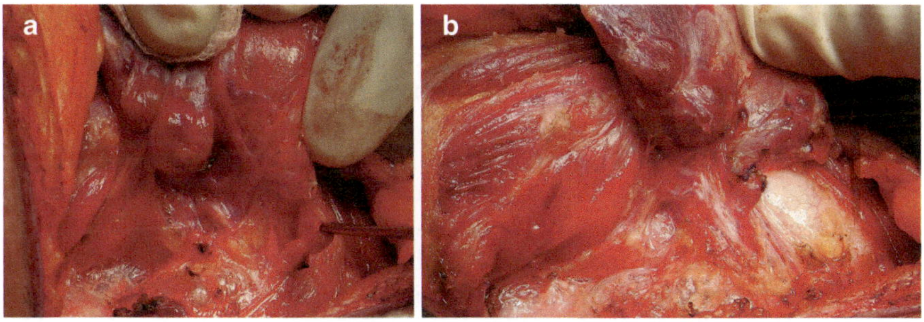

Fig. 6.21 Inferior parathyroid glands

Fig. 6.22 Ectopic thyroid rests

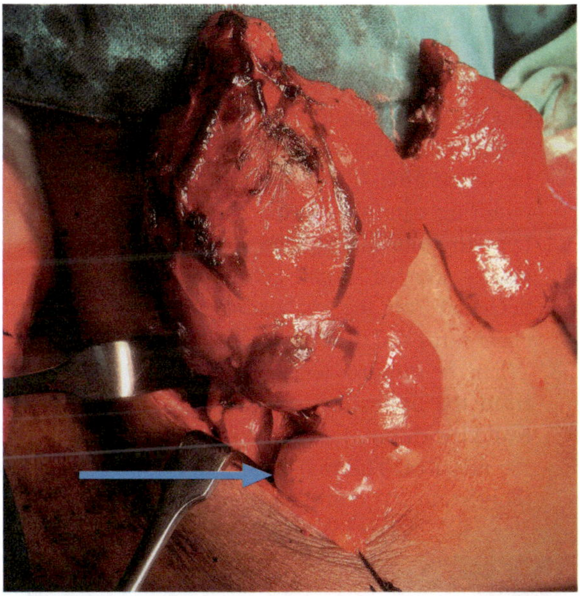

nidus for primary mediastinal goitres with separate blood vessels. CT of the neck demonstrates the extent of mediastinal extension and a detailed analysis of axial, sagittal, and coronal views is done before the operation. The majority of mediastinal goitres are direct extensions of the lower pole of the lobe to the superior mediastinum and thyroid tissue seldom receives blood supply from mediastinal vessels. The RLN is usually preserved in the normal course in the neck. Rarely do nodules from the posterior aspect grow to the posterior mediastinum changing the course of RLN. Primary mediastinal goitres are rare but develop from ectopic thyroid tissue and derive their blood supply from mediastinal vessels.

Mediastinal extension beyond the aortic arch reaching up to carina, and primary mediastinal goitre are indications for sternotomy. Recurrent goitre with mediastinal extension also may require sternotomy possibly due to vascular adhesions.

The thyroid is mobilised by dividing the superior pole, middle thyroid veins, and other veins in the neck. The dissection of the contralateral lobe is difficult since the trachea is invariably shifted to the opposite side. Release of SCM from the strap muscles facilitates retraction of the muscles. Langenbeck retractor is placed to retract the SCM exposing the lateral aspect of the lobe and further vascular connections divided. Gentle traction given on the cervical portion of goitre with good retraction further exposes the mediastinal part. Blunt dissection is done on the mediastinal gently with fingers and a combination of traction and finger dissection delivers the goitre in the neck wound. Overzealous traction or finger dissection should be avoided since ensuing bleeding is troublesome (Fig. 6.23a, b).

26. The lobe is lifted off the bed by separating it from the trachea by energy sources since the thyroid receives blood supply from tracheal vessels also. The superior pole is held with a Babcock's forceps and dissection is continued in cricothyroid space. The plane is usually avascular but may encounter difficulty in thyroid cancers with extra-thyroid spread and concurrent thyroiditis (Fig. 6.24a–c).
27. Thyroid lobe is dissected off the trachea with energy sources. There are vascular connections to the thyroid gland from tracheal and oesophageal vessels requiring careful control. These vessels assume considerable significance in hyperthyroidism and need careful control. Indiscriminate use of high-intensity energy sources should be avoided to preserve tracheal integrity. The lobe is detached from the trachea medially up to the midline. Isthmus is lifted of tracheal rings and the opposite lobe is reached.
28. When hemithyroidectomy is planned the lobe and isthmus are detached from the opposite lobe with sharp dissection. Bleeding vessels are controlled with bipolar diathermy taking precautions not to burn the trachea or the muscles. Thermal injury can induce fibrosis and can cause difficulty in mobilisation if completion thyroidectomy is necessary. The pyramidal lobe

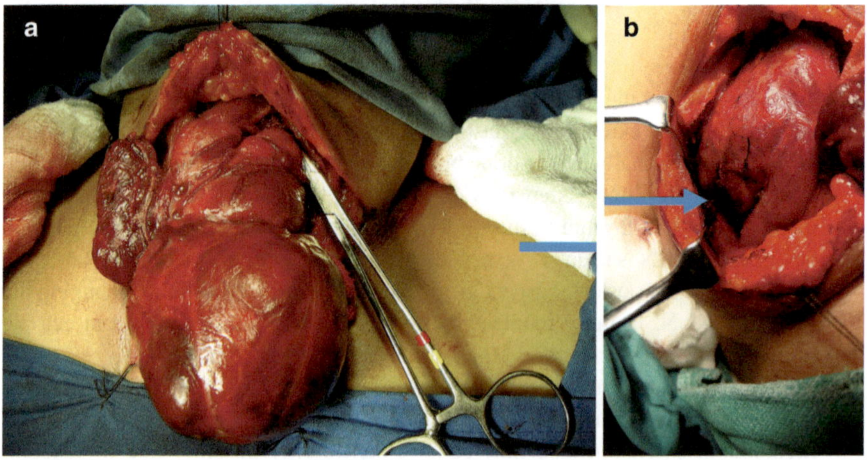

Fig. 6.23 Dissection of retrosternal extension

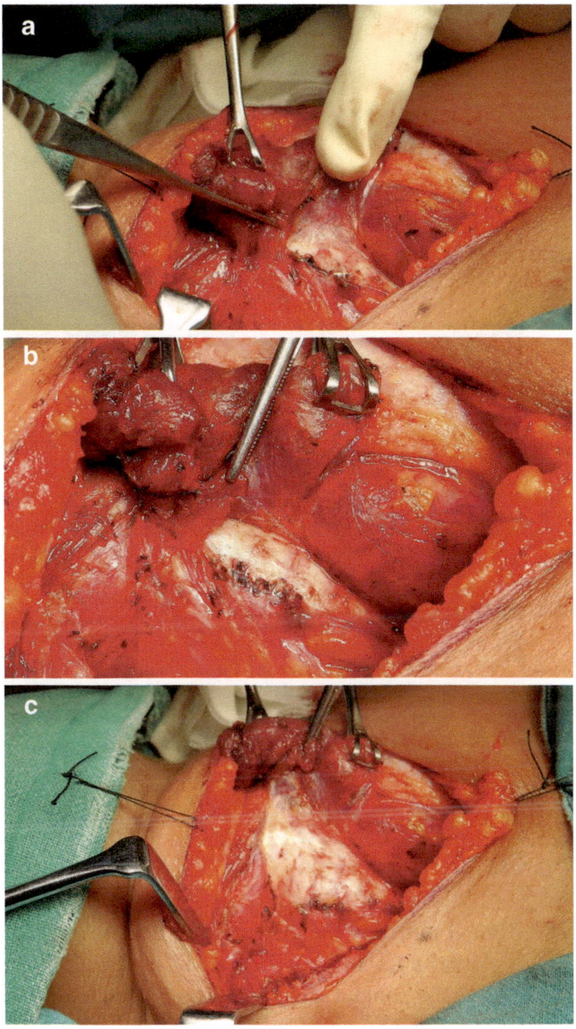

Fig. 6.24 Mobilisation of right lobe from trachea

and thyroglossal tract are also removed when found attached to the index lobe. Attempting to mobilise the opposite lobe for inspection is not advisable as it induces fibrosis which will tell upon completion thyroidectomy when required (Fig. 6.25).

29. The opposite lobe is treated in a similar fashion. Exposure of the opposite lobe is commenced by lifting the strap muscle. The lateral aspect of the lobe is mobilised from strap muscles and sternocleidomastoid muscles and steadied with a retractor. The surgeon may have to move to the opposite side for the latter part of the procedure since the course of RLN is better visible from the index side (Fig. 6.26a–d).

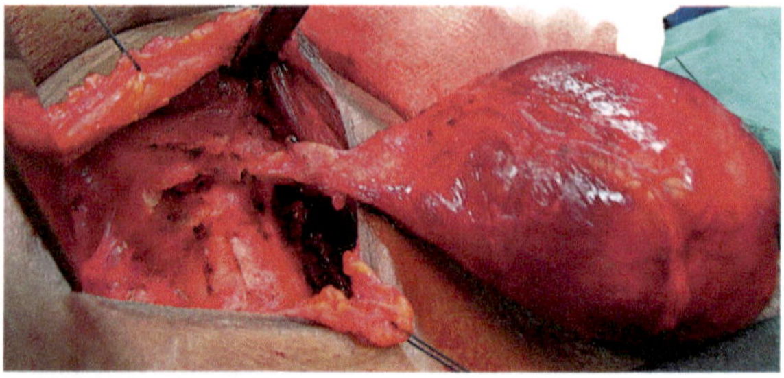

Fig. 6.25 Right hemithyroidectomy

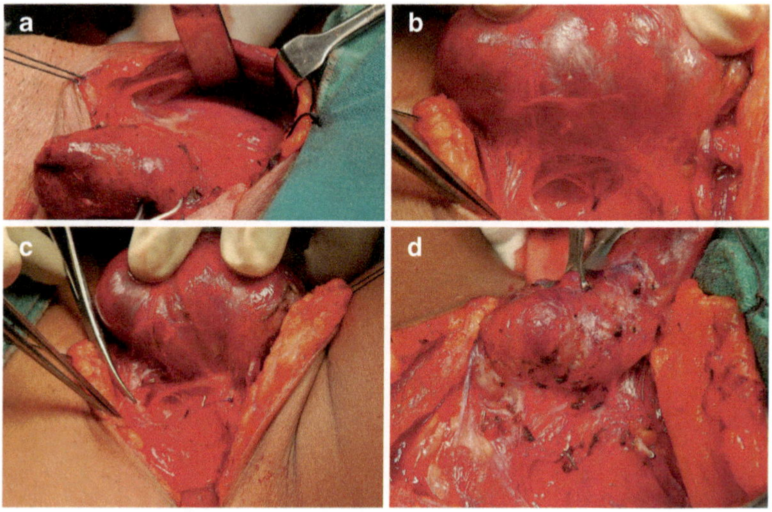

Fig. 6.26 Left lobe dissection

30. After completing the dissection of both lobes, the pyramidal lobe and the thyroglossal tract are removed along with the thyroid gland. The Thyro-glossal tract may contain glandular tissue and is followed up to the hyoid bone (Fig. 6.27a, b).
31. The entire specimen is removed and inspected closely for incidental removal of the parathyroid gland. If any suspicious tissue is found a bit is removed for frozen section studies and confirmed tissue is sliced to 1 mm slices and implanted to pouches of sternomastoid muscle (four to five slices in one pouch). The opening in the muscle is closed with clips or sutures.
32. The thyroid bed is inspected for bleeding points and integrity of parathyroid glands. A Langenbeck retractor displaces muscles laterally and the assistant holds the trachea medially to expose the thyroid bed on one side. The RLN and parathyroid glands are inspected. A saline wash of the thyroid bed helps to identify bleeding vessels. The anaesthesiologist performs Valsalva manoeuvre once or twice for 30 s applying 30-cm positive-end expiratory pressure to iden-

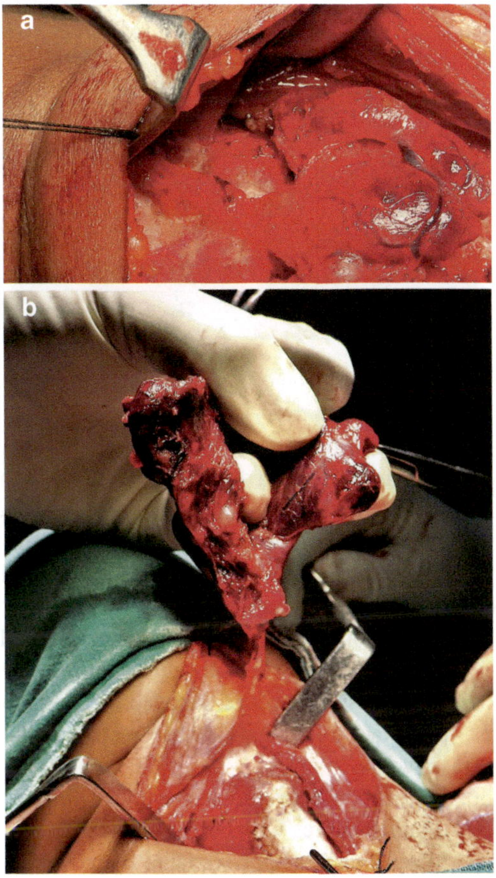

Fig. 6.27 Dissection of the Thyroglossal tract

tify potential bleeding points. The use of intraoperative Valsalva manoeuvre has questionable benefits but is found beneficial in personal practice. Haemostasis is ensured by judicious use of diathermy after ensuring the site and course of laryngeal nerves and parathyroid glands. Sites to be cautiously inspected include superior polar vessel stumps, the surface of the trachea, and the cut end of any muscles (Fig. 6.28a, b).

33. Colour and appearance of the parathyroid glands should be inspected. Dusky-looking or obviously dark parathyroid glands are subjected to a knife test using a number 11 blade. Active bleeding on pricking with the blade ensures vascularity of the nerve. A traumatised gland may be tense with a drop of blood and the knife prick helps to decompress it.
34. Closure of the wound is equally important since the scar is always visible and seldom concealed by most of the dress codes. Traditionally wound drains are kept following thyroidectomy. But reviews failed to establish advantages favouring routine use of wound drains. There was no difference found between

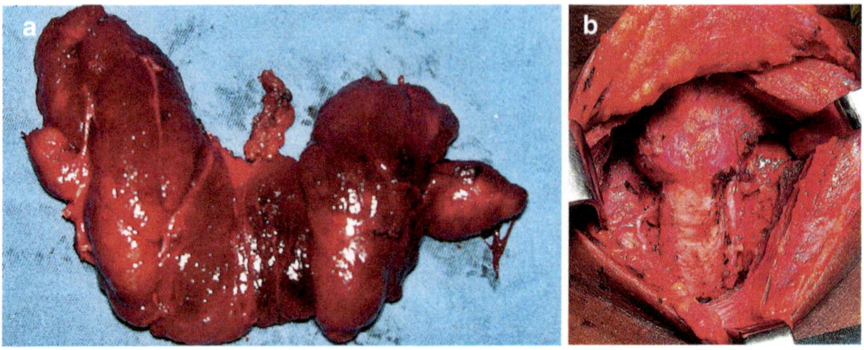

Fig. 6.28 (**a**) Inspection of thyroidectomy specimen and (**b**) Thyroid bed

routine drainage and no drainage with regard to the frequency of postoperative hematoma/seroma following thyroidectomy [2, 3]. But drain may be placed based on the surgeon's judgment considering features such as retrosternal extension, large volume goitre, and lymph node dissections [4]. In case a suction drain is kept a single limb is inserted just lateral to the end of the main incision taking care of the external jugular vein. Adequate care is taken to keep the end of the drain away from the thyroid bed to protect the RLN and parathyroid glands from suction injuries (Fig. 6.29a–d).

35. The investing layer of the deep fascia is closed by interrupted sutures using 3-0 polyglactin filaments. Care should be taken to avoid injuries to anterior jugular veins.
36. Platysma is approximated with subcutaneous tissue using 3-0 polyglactin continuous sutures with buried knots.
37. Skin edges are approximated by running subcuticular sutures using monofilament absorbable suture materials like 4-0 Poliglecaprone 25 (Monocryl).
38. Occlusive wound dressings are applied.

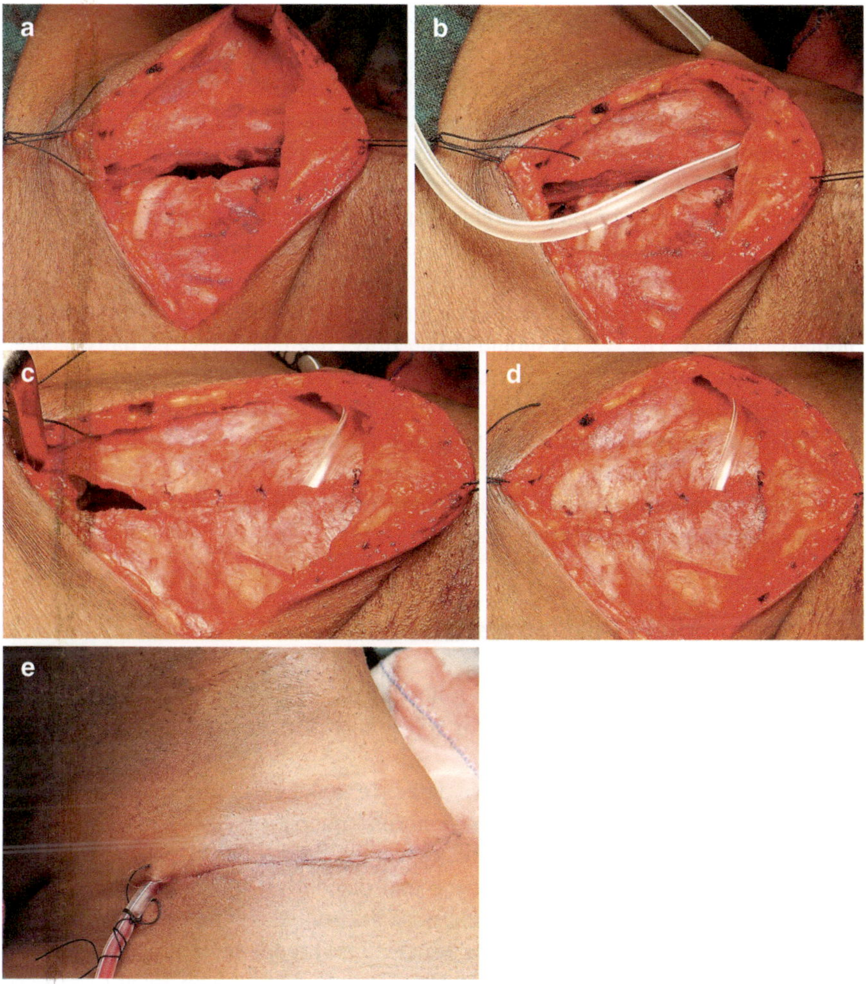

Fig. 6.29 Closure

6.2 Goitres with Mediastinal Extension

The goitres with mediastinal extensions derive their blood supply from regular blood vessels supplying the gland. Successful mobilisation of the mediastinal portion is almost always possible through a cervical approach by careful dissection.

Dissection of this portion is done after the division of all known blood vessels on both sides. The main surgeon preferably stands on the side of the mediastinal extension and the first assistant holds the goitre medially. The second assistant retracts the lower third of muscles laterally. To facilitate better exposure the course of RLN is followed towards mediastinum with combination blunt and sharp dissection using bipolar diathermy. The vessels should be carefully coagulated since partially secured vessels retract to the mediastinum leading to bleeding. The first assistant who holds the goitre medially can exert judicious traction while the lateral dissection is continued and the goitre is delivered to the neck. It is not advisable to perform blind finger dissection.

Median sternotomy is rarely required and common indications are malignancy, primary goitres, and recurrent goitres.

6.3 Immediate Post-operative Period

Direct laryngoscopy is recommended following removal of endotracheal tube.

Close monitoring of the patient for 6 h following completion of procedure is recommended.

Patients who were detected to have defective vocal cord movement are closely observed for 24 h even if found to have normal phonation and respiration. These patients are at risk of aspiration of food, especially fluids.

Excessive pain, tightness of the neck and discomfort to breath may be early symptoms of haematoma formation and warrants immediate intervention.

Toxic crisis is infrequent now due to adequate preoperative preparations. But there are occasional patients with refractory Graves' disease who are at risk of crisis. These patients warrant close monitoring since patient may crash suddenly. It is advisable to estimate serum free T4 and T3 after operation.

Serum corrected calcium estimation after 6 h of completion surgery is routine in our institution and a drop of 1 mg or more from preoperative level is a predictor of hypocalcaemia. The sensitivity of this test is very low but cheap compared to intraoperative iPTH estimation. Majority of patients are free of pain and do not require analgesics on second postoperative day.

Management of major complications are explained in subsequent chapters.

6.4 Discharge from Hospital

Most of patients are fit for discharge after 24 h if patient is asymptomatic and serum corrected calcium level remain in normal ranges. There is no need for peri-operative or prophylactic antibiotic administration. Patient is suggested mild analgesics like paracetamol and advised to undertake routine household activities. Patient is suggested routine shower bath after 48 h but the operated area is moped dry but should not apply any cosmetics in and around the incision site. Routine application of topical antibiotic cream is not recommended. Thyroxine supplementation even for benign goitres are avoided since histological surprises are not unusual. Iodine restricted diet is recommended in patients who had preoperative diagnosis of thyroid carcinoma.

Patients who got discharged after 24 h with a stable general condition and serum calcium level are advised to keep a watch on manifestation of symptoms due to hypocalcaemia. (Unexplained tiredness, tinkling sensation in fingertips and circumoral region, muscle spasm and breathing difficulty.) Patients are advised to report to nearest hospital for emergency management or to index hospital for further management.

All patients are reviewed after 7 days for appraisal wound site and serum calcium level. Rare patients may develop delayed biochemical hypocalcaemia.

6.5 Postoperative Management of Benign Thyroid Diseases

Thyroidectomy is performed for benign diseases such as nodular goitre, toxic nodular goitre and Graves' disease. Diagnostic hemithyroidectomy and total thyroidectomy are performed with for patients with suspicious cytology.

6.6 General Instructions

Majority of patients are discharged 48 h after operation and are advised to undertake all routine activities for personal needs at home. There is no need for bedrest at home but those who had symptomatic hypocalcaemia are advised to avoid standing or walking for long time since many patients may develop neuromuscular symptoms. Many patients have misconception regarding taking baths or wetting operated site. Epithelisation had been completed within 48 h and so migration of bacteria is unlikely. Topical antiseptic cream is not advisable since it has no proven efficacy and forms a crest on the incision site.

Patients who have compromised laryngeal function are instructed to undertake voice rest, and proper swallowing techniques. They are advised to avoid gulping fluids and it is better to mix fluids with solid foods during meal time. This may help them to avoid aspiration to larynx and further related complications.

Those who are on calcium supplementation are instructed to comply properly with drug regimen in dose and time schedule.

Patients are encouraged to undertake all routine activities 7–10 days after the operation which shall meet their family, social and office needs.

Thyroid hormone supplementation is not started when the patients are discharged after operation. Probability of incidental thyroid cancers is 5–10% and increased TSH level help them to undergo early iodine ablation when required. Since the half life of natural thyroxine is also 4–5 days, clinical manifestations of hypothyroidism are rare.

Patients who underwent diagnostic hemithyroidectomy with negative biopsy report for cancer shall be kept under observation. Euthyroid status is maintained in approximately 80% of patients and first screening is done 1 month after operation. If the patient is clinically asymptomatic and free T4 and TSH level are well maintained in normal ranges thyroxine supplementation is not indicated. Patients need a closer follow up when TSH level show an upward trend or lymphocytic thyroiditis was present in excised thyroid tissue.

Patients who underwent total or near total thyroidectomy require hormone supplementation. The hormone was isolated as early as 1900 but derivative was synthesised in 1927 by Charles Robert Harington and George Barger. Since then, levothyroxine is one of the widely used molecules. But the schedule and dosage were mostly established in hypothyroidism due to causes other than thyroidectomy.

Requirement of levothyroxine following thyroidectomy varies greatly among patients and is influenced by age, sex, BMI, and body surface area. Various formulae were tried incorporating these factors [5].

Traditionally levothyroxine is started as 1.6 μg/kg body weight but many patients require dosage adjustment to achieve euthyroid status. In routine clinical practice levothyroxine is started as standard regimen of 100 μg daily for an adult weighing about 60 kg with no cardiac ailments. Patients properly instructed to take tablets in the morning before food for proper absorption and other medications like proton pump inhibitors (PPI) are not consumed simultaneously. Patients are reviewed after 1 month for thyroid function studies. TSH needs longer time for normalisation and the dose is adjusted based on FT4 values. Majority of patients become euthyroid by the first review itself.

References

1. Tomoda C, Kitano H, Uruno T, Takamura Y, Ito Y, Miya A, Kobayashi K, Matsuzuka F, Amino N, Kuma K, Miyauchi A. Transcutaneous iodine absorption in adult patients with thyroid cancer disinfected with povidone-iodine at operation. Thyroid. 2005;15(6):600–3.
2. Sanabria A, Carvalho AL, Silver CE, Rinaldo A, Shaha AR, Kowalski LP, Ferlito A. Routine drainage after thyroid surgery—a meta-analysis. J Surg Oncol. 2007;96:273–80.
3. Samraj K, Gurusamy KS. Wound drains following thyroid surgery. Cochrane Database Syst Rev. 2007;2007(4):CD006099. https://doi.org/10.1002/14651858.CD006099.pub2.
4. Woods RS, Woods JF, Duignan ES, Timon C. Systematic review and meta-analysis of wound drains after thyroid surgery. Br J Surg. 2014;101(5):446–56.
5. Miccoli P, Materazzi G, Rossi L. Levothyroxine therapy in thyrodectomized patients. Front Endocrinol (Lausanne). 2021;11:626268. https://doi.org/10.3389/fendo.2020.626268.

Central Compartment Lymph Node Dissection

7

Riju Ramachandran, C. Gopalakrishnan Nair, and Pradeep Jacob

Papillary thyroid cancer metastasises frequently through lymph nodes and the central compartment is considered the first nodal station. Lymph nodes in the central compartment are seldom detected preoperatively on ultrasound imaging. Central compartment lymph node dissection (CCD) carries an increased risk of injury to RLN and parathyroid glands even in trained hands. Prophylactic CCD was recommended for papillary thyroid cancers but the overall impact on the outcome of the procedure is debated. Prophylactic central compartment dissection is not routinely performed for stage 1 and 2 papillary thyroid cancers. CCD is always done therapeutically and also along with MRND for clearance of all nodal stations.

American Thyroid Association surgery working group came out with a consensus statement regarding the boundaries of the central compartment in 2009 [1]. The central compartment is bounded superiorly by the hyoid bone, laterally by the carotid arteries, anteriorly by the superficial layer of the deep cervical fascia, and posteriorly by the deep layer of the deep cervical fascia. Lymph nodes are scattered in the prelaryngeal region, peri-thyroid region, pre-tracheal station, and paratracheal region.

The sensitivity of preoperative imaging to detect central compartment nodes is very low. The air-filled trachea and oesophagus interfere with ultrasound imaging. Contrast-enhanced CT is superior in detecting central compartment nodes. During surgical procedures, lymph nodes >1 cm size and the presence of adhesions are features indicating metastasis.

The pre-laryngeal and peri-thyroid nodes are harvested along with thyroidectomy. Paratracheal nodes are scattered on the lateral and anterior sides of trachea

C. G. Nair (✉)
Professor of Surgery, Endocrine Surgery Division, Amrita Institute of Medical Sciences and Research Centre, Kochi, Kerala, India

R. Ramachandran · P. Jacob
Department of Surgery, AIMS, Kochi, Kochi, Kerala, India

C. G. Nair, S. J. Abraham (eds.), *Surgical Management of Thyroid and Parathyroid Diseases*, https://doi.org/10.1007/978-981-97-3774-1_7

and the chain extends to the superior mediastinum. The paratracheal lymph nodes have variable but close distribution around recurrent laryngeal nerves and dissection is technically difficult.

The inferior parathyroid glands are usually embedded in the perithyroidal soft tissue close to the lower pole of lobes and are in risk for direct injury and vascular damage.

Steps of procedure:

1. Central compartment dissection is commenced after the division of the superior thyroid artery. The lobe is rotated medially exposing perithyroidal and paratracheal stations (Fig. 7.1).
2. The lobe is retracted medially by the first assistant exposing the lateral aspect of the larynx and trachea. The enlarged peri-thyroid nodes interfere with the identification of recurrent laryngeal nerve. The RLN is preferably identified before it crosses the inferior thyroid artery since pre-laryngeal divisions when present may be splayed by the perithyroidal lymph nodes (Fig. 7.2). More frequently the enlarged nodes cover the RLN and the nerve is exposed by gentle dissection (Fig. 7.3).
3. During mobilisation of the lobe of the thyroid, the peri-thyroid soft tissue, paratracheal area, and pre-tracheal area are inspected for enlarged lymph nodes. Lymph nodes larger than 1 cm are significant and warrant dissection. Frozen section biopsy is not always helpful since micro-metastases (<2 mm) are not always detected. The characteristic blue nodes are not routinely found (Fig. 7.4).
4. The RLN is traced from the distal portion towards the root of the neck using a combination of sharp and blunt dissection. The first assistant holds the lobe steady while a third assistant on the left side of the surgeon retracts the strap muscles laterally exposing the central compartment. The use of bipolar micro tips under low-intensity power is advisable to safeguard the RLN and parathyroid glands. Indiscriminate usage of diathermy is not recommended even after the course of nerve is defined.
5. The trunk of RLN is traced towards the mediastinum by lifting the soft tissue above it. A curved haemostat is inserted in the direction of the course of nerve

Fig. 7.1 Exposure of perithyroidal lymph nodes

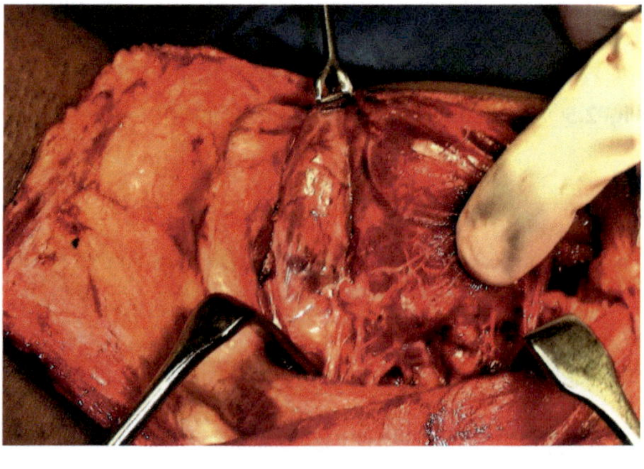

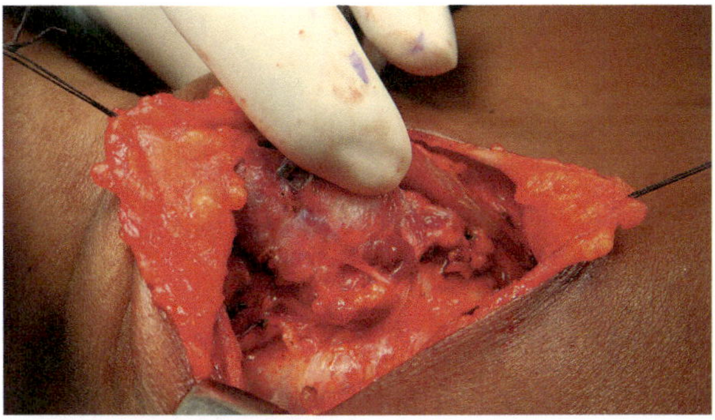

Fig. 7.2 Pre-laryngeal divisions of right RLN and lymph nodes

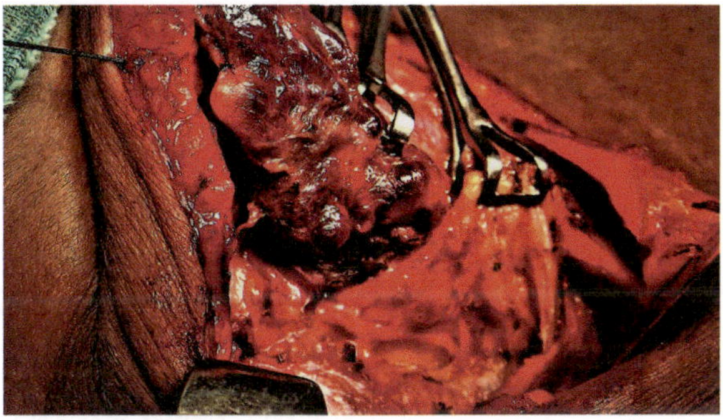

Fig. 7.3 Cervical portion RLN is dissected

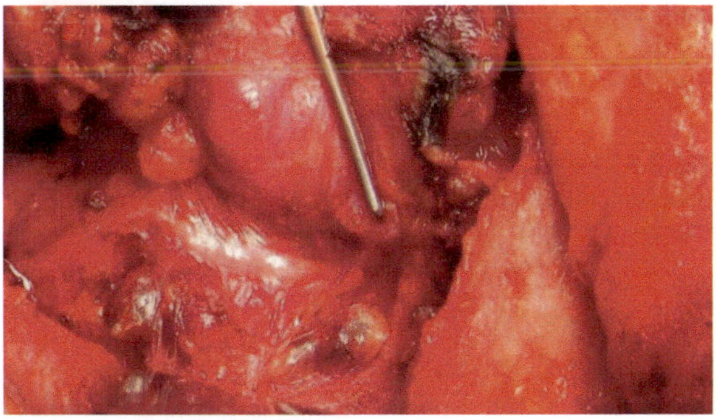

Fig. 7.4 Characteristic blue node in central compartment

under the vision and the soft tissue is divided linear fashion exposing the cervical course of RLN (Fig. 7.5).

6. Soft tissue between the RLN and the carotid artery is hooked up using a DeBakey and removed. The tissue plane is usually avascular and so better dissected with scissors rather than diathermy to avoid thermal injury of RLN. The cervical course of RLN is exposed on both sides (Figs. 7.5 and 7.6).
7. The carotid artery may course anteriorly over the trachea on the right side. On such occasions, the common carotid artery is mobilised preserving the vagal trunk and held on a vascular loop for adequate exposure (Figs. 7.7 and 7.8).

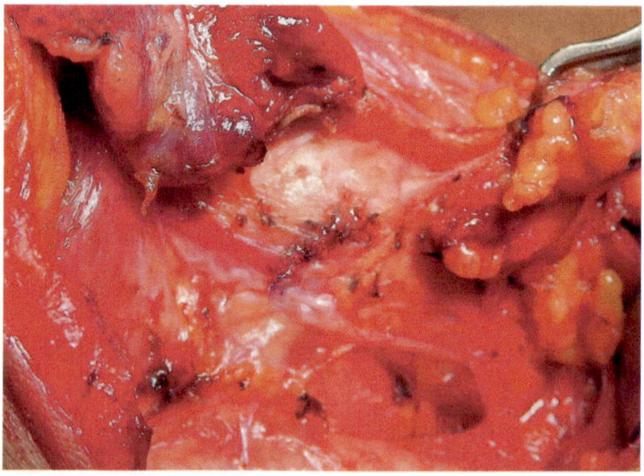

Fig. 7.5 Full length of right RLN dissected

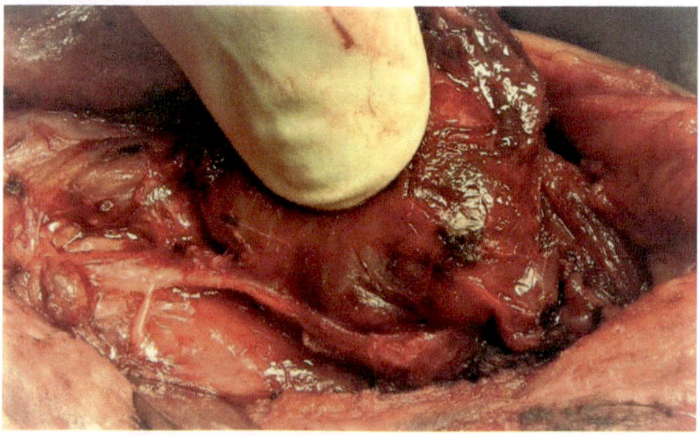

Fig. 7.6 Left RLN adherent to thyroid with nodes being exposed

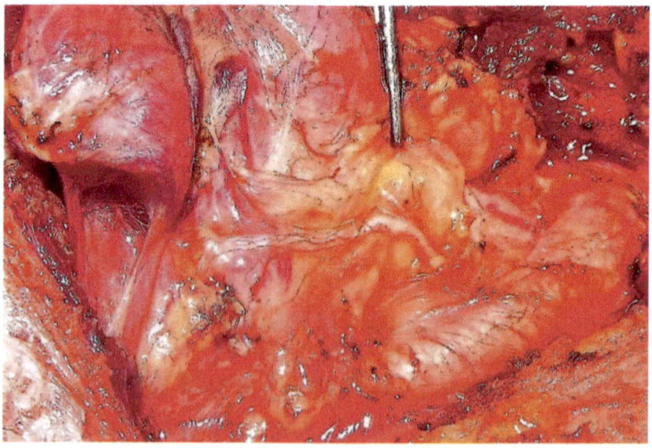

Fig. 7.7 Right side dissection of carotid artery over rides trachea

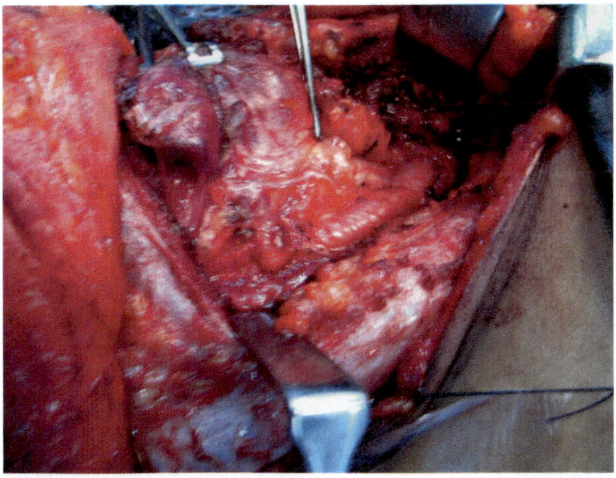

Fig. 7.8 Right side carotid artery riding over trachea

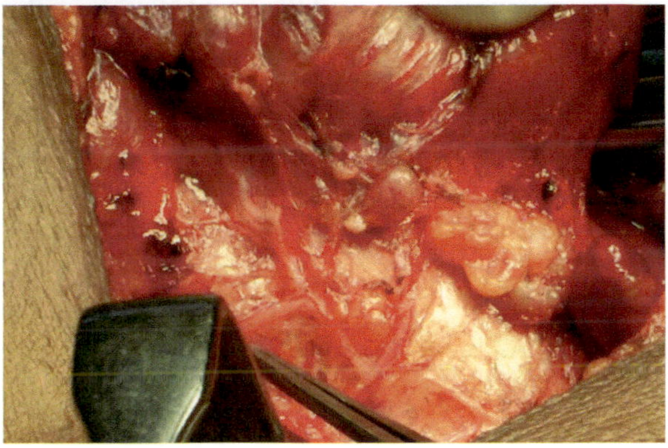

Fig. 7.9 Right side CCD in progress

8. Inferior parathyroid glands are inconstant in position and so localisation may be difficult. The parathyroid artery from the inferior division of the ITA may show a road map.
9. The inferior thyroid veins are secured cautiously since the vessel may retract to the superior mediastinum and bleeding may be troublesome. Lymph nodes in paratracheal, peritracheal, and perithyroidal stations are harvested as a single bunch (Figs. 7.9 and 7.10).
10. The pre-tracheal and paratracheal lymph nodes are removed en-block with the isthmus preserving the parathyroid glands (Figs. 7.11, 7.12, and 7.13).
11. The parathyroid glands are inspected prior to the closure of the wound.
12. Wound closure is done routinely as discussed earlier but the placement of 12 F suction drain is routine.

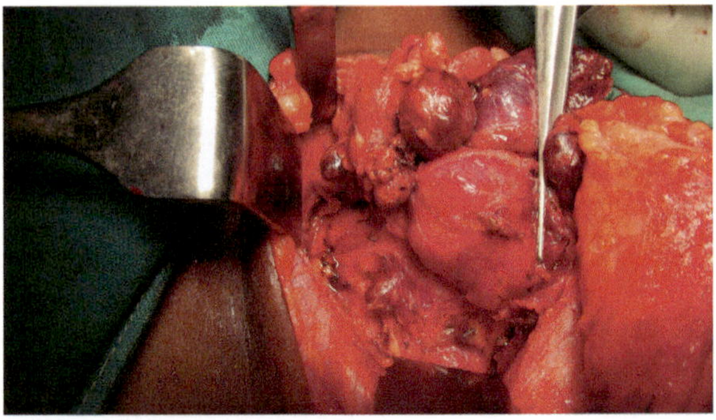

Fig. 7.10 Left side CCD in progress

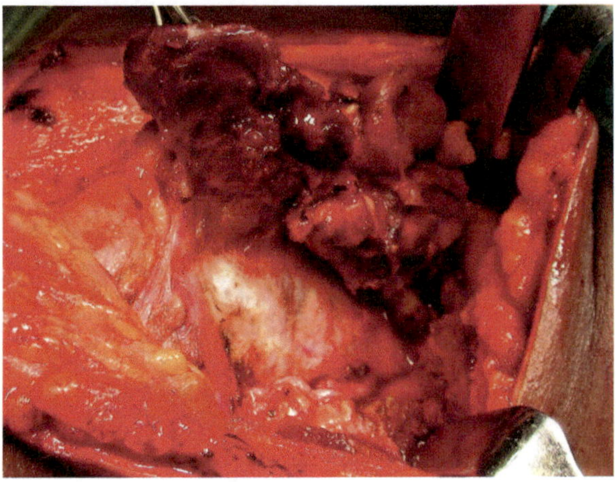

Fig. 7.11 Right paratracheal nodes dissected

Fig. 7.12 Bilateral dissection completed

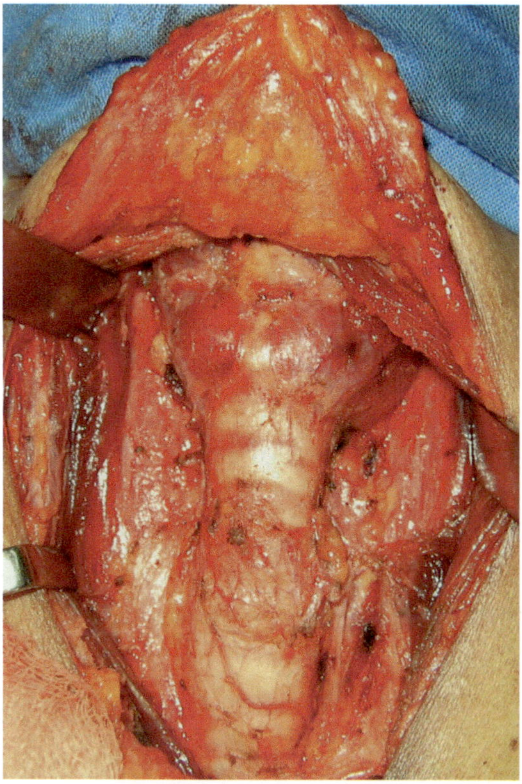

Fig. 7.13 Thyroid with central compartment nodes

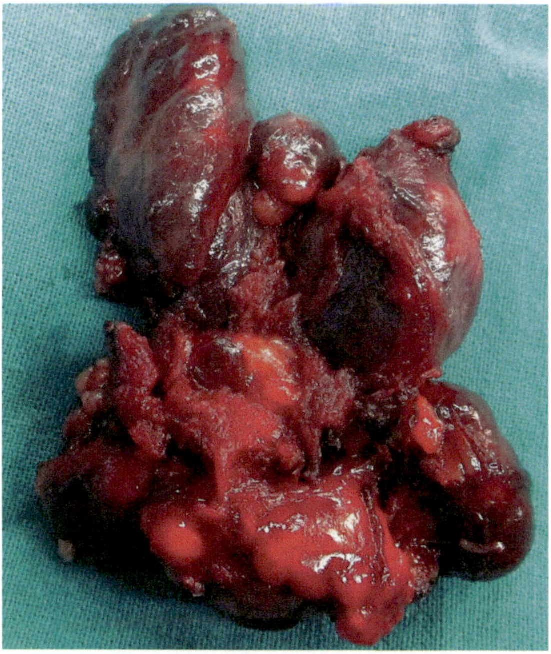

Reference

1. American Thyroid Association Surgery Working Group. American Association of Endocrine Surgeons; American Academy of Otolaryngology-Head and Neck Surgery; American Head and Neck Society, Carty SE, Cooper DS, Doherty GM, et al. Consensus statement on the terminology and classification of central neck dissection for thyroid cancer. Thyroid. 2009;19:1153–8. https://doi.org/10.1089/thy.2009.0159.

Modified Segment Oriented Cervical Lymph Node Dissection for Thyroid Cancer

8

C. Gopalakrishnan Nair and Misha J. C. Babu

8.1 Introduction

The commonest mode of locoregional spread of thyroid cancer is to the regional nodal basin. The frequency of lymph node metastases varies among different pathological types of thyroid cancers. The lymph node metastases are very common in papillary thyroid cancers but infrequent in follicular thyroid cancers. Noguchi (1970) considered the pattern of lymph node spread was systematic with the paratracheal or central compartment being the first nodal station. But the pattern of lymph node spread is not always systematic and skip metastases are frequent. The extend of nodal disease is generally limited to nodes below the hyoid level and the submandibular area is usually spared. The lymph node dissection is known as segment-oriented selective neck dissection removing lymph nodes in Level IV, Level III, and Level II-A stations. Dissection extends to Level V station when lymph nodes are found along with the transverse cervical artery. Level II-B stations rarely harbour metastatic nodes except for contiguous spread from the II-B area. Removal of nodes in Level II-B is advisable when metastatic nodes are found in Level II-A stations Level VI nodes are removed along with thyroidectomy when neck dissection is performed concurrently. Level I nodes are seldom removed.

The incision should be planned carefully since cosmesis is very important. The phrenic nerve and spinal accessory nerve are of paramount importance in cervical block dissection. These nerves are at risk when dissection is done for metastatic lymph nodes with perinodal spread.

C. G. Nair (✉)
Professor of Surgery, Endocrine Surgery Division, Amrita Institute of Medical Sciences and Research Centre, Kochi, Kerala, India

M. J. C. Babu
Department of General Surgery, AIMS, Kochi, Kochi, Kerala, India

C. G. Nair, S. J. Abraham (eds.), *Surgical Management of Thyroid and Parathyroid Diseases*, https://doi.org/10.1007/978-981-97-3774-1_8

Generally, sternomastoid muscles, internal jugular veins, and spinal accessory nerves are preserved. The internal jugular vein is removed when nodes are adherent to the vessel wall or when luminal thrombosis is suspected. The sternocleidomastoid muscle is always preserved but occasionally divided for better exposure of Level II-B station.

Meticulous removal of lymph nodes is of great importance in medullary thyroid cancers since surgical treatment is the only option with curative intent. Re-entry to a previously operated field for removal of a recurrence carries a higher risk of injury to major structures.

The thoracic duct is an important structure and should be identified and preserved on the left side. Metastatic nodes are occasionally found posterior to the terminal portion of the internal jugular vein and dissection of these nodes should be done with caution. The thoracic duct has variable relation to IJV and is at risk especially when perinodal adhesions are present. Three vital structures of paramount importance in the field of operation are the spinal accessory nerve, phrenic nerve, and thoracic duct. Injury of any of these structures leads to lasting major morbidity and could be even fatal.

8.2 The Steps of Surgical Procedure

The procedure is combined with total thyroidectomy if spread to lateral lymph node is confirmed or as an additional procedure when lymph node recurrences are confirmed during the follow-up period. The procedure is always done under general anaesthesia with endotracheal intubation. The patient is positioned supine with a gel pad under the shoulder and a padded ring to steady the head. The shoulder roll and ring are adjusted for maximum exposure but an overenthusiastic extension of the cervical spine should be avoided. The neck is turned to the opposite side for better exposure.

Incision:

1. Lateral extension of the traditional thyroidectomy incision towards the anterior border of SCM with a curvy-linear extension along the line of its posterior border for 1 or 2 cm yields adequate exposure and acceptable cosmetics. Vertical ascending incisions are better avoided since the cosmesis is badly affected (Figs. 8.1, 8.2, 8.3, 8.4, and 8.5).
2. Skin flap is made to reach hyoid bone in midline and angle of mandible on the index side (Figs. 8.6 and 8.7).
3. Lower flap is made to reach the clavicle exposing the insertion of SCM. Careful haemostasis is ensured since there is a wide raw area. The lower flap dissection extends laterally beyond the SCM on the side of lymph node dissection.
4. After completing total thyroidectomy and central compartment dissection a wet gauze is placed over the thyroid bed (Fig. 8.8).
5. For the initial steps of the dissection the surgeon may remain on the right side of the patient when the procedure is coupled with total thyroidectomy. (Right-handed person.) But authors prefer the surgeon on the side of dissection and

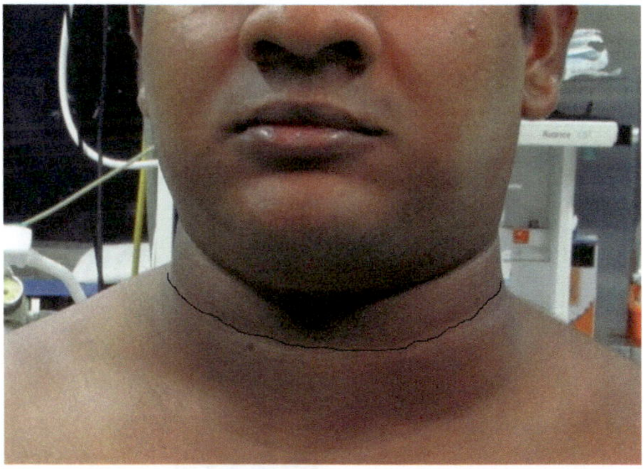

Fig. 8.1 Designing incision before anaesthesia

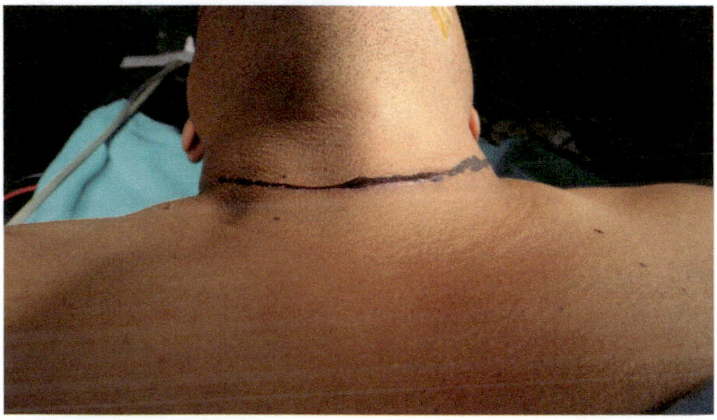

Fig. 8.2 Patient positioned with preplanned incision

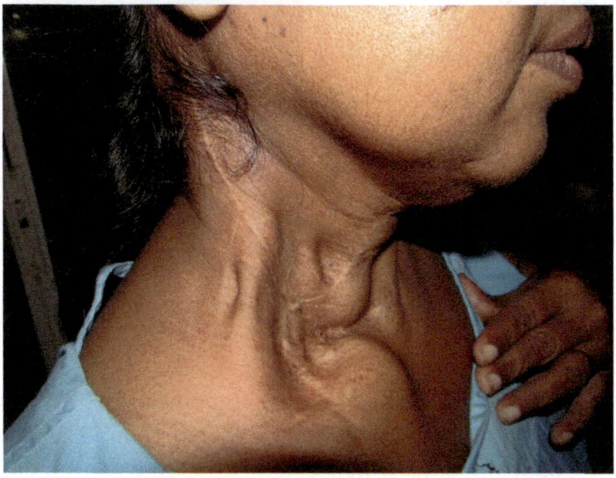

Fig. 8.3 Bad scar of a neck dissection

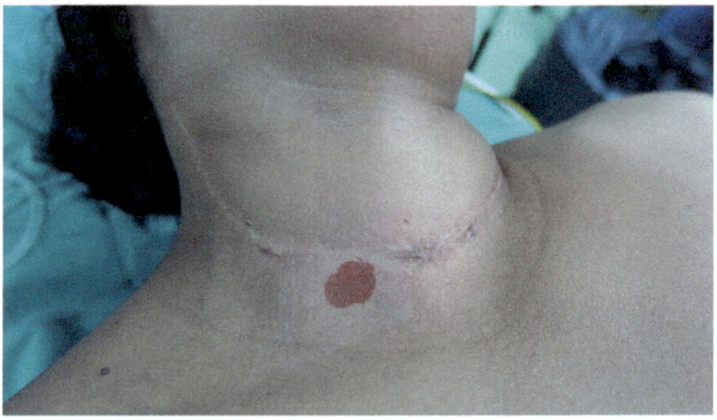

Fig. 8.4 The extension of the lateral end of incision is not necessary

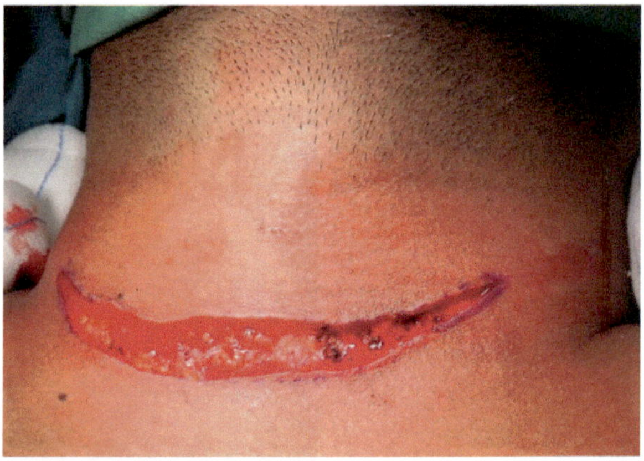

Fig. 8.5 Incision made

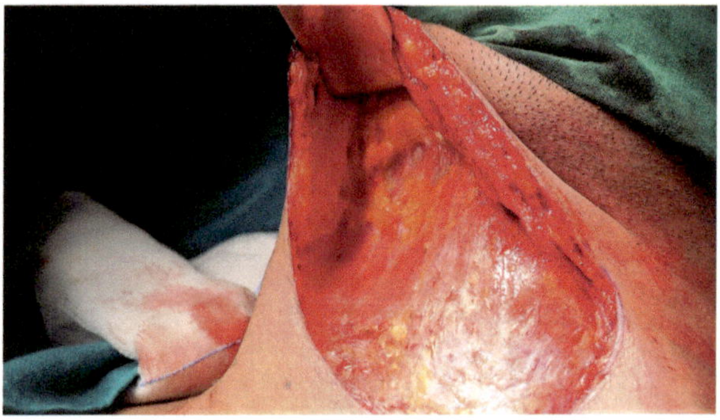

Fig. 8.6 Skin flap

the first assistant stands on the other side. A third assistant when joining the team stands on the side of the surgeon. The scrub nurse shall move to the opposite side which enables the free movements of the surgeon and third assistant.

6. The strap muscle is stretched medially holding it with tissue holding forceps while the SCM is stretched laterally. This manure exposes an oblique line in the deep fascia between the two sets of muscles (Figs. 8.7 and 8.9).

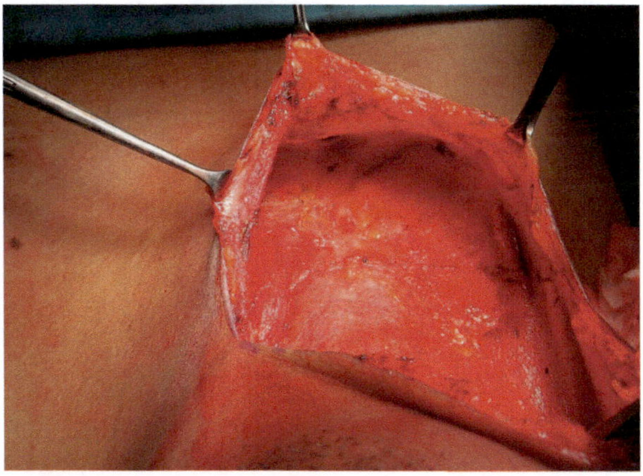

Fig. 8.7 Skin flap

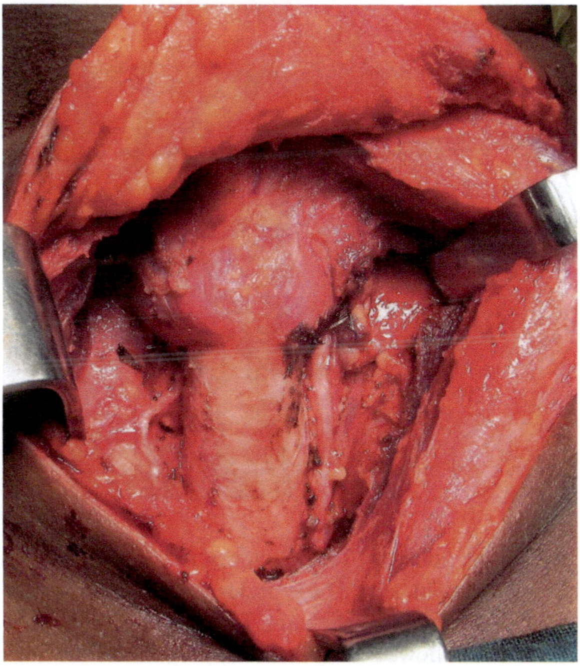

Fig. 8.8 Total thyroidectomy completed

7. These strap muscles are separated from sternomastoid muscle using sharp dissection. The monopolar diathermy is used with caution to avoid injury to carotid sheath structures. The dissection starts in the lower neck since the carotid sheath is relatively at a deeper plane. Blood vessels encountered during the dissection are secured effectively since they may be draining directly to IJV. The first assistant holds medial retraction preferably holding the tissues with wet gauze. Langenbeck retractor is judiciously placed to retract the sternocleidomastoid muscle to expose the carotid sheath.

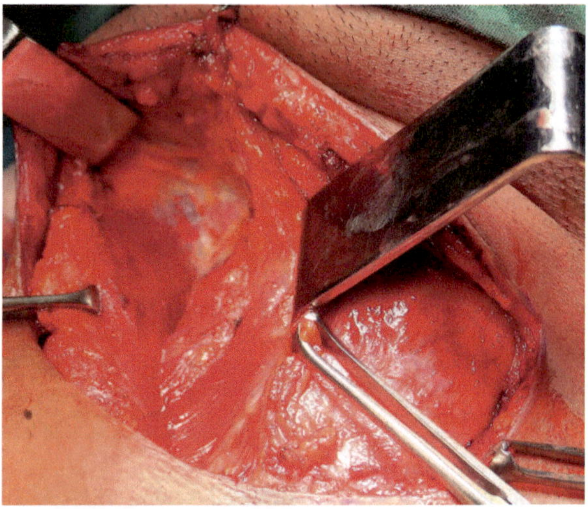

Fig. 8.9 Incision of deep fascia between strap muscles and SCM

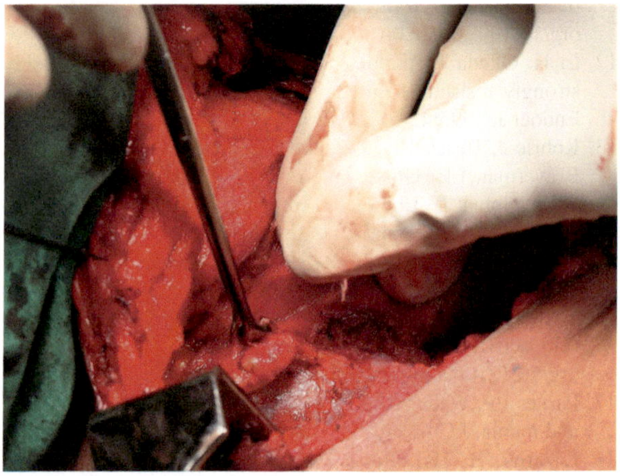

Fig. 8.10 Lymph nodes on the anterior surface of IJV

8. Lymph nodes are found anterior to IJV at close to the point of entry of the superior thyroid vein. These nodes may assume large size and have to be dissected free for exposing the vein (Fig. 8.10).
9. IJV is followed towards the upper third of the neck where the carotid sheath is relatively superficial. The upper third of IJV is exposed with and digastric muscle crossing the vein (Fig. 8.11).
10. Mobilization of IJV continues towards the lower part of the neck where the carotid sheath is placed at a deeper plane. The omohyoid muscle crosses the IJV anteriorly and for exposure, the muscle is divided. The muscle is lifted from the IJV by gentle blunt dissection and divided using bipolar diathermy (Figs. 8.12 and 8.13). IJV, carotid artery, and vagus nerve are exposed in full length (Fig. 8.14).

    The soft tissue around the IJV is dissected to skeletonise the vessel. The dissection starts on the anterior surface initially and continues to the lateral and

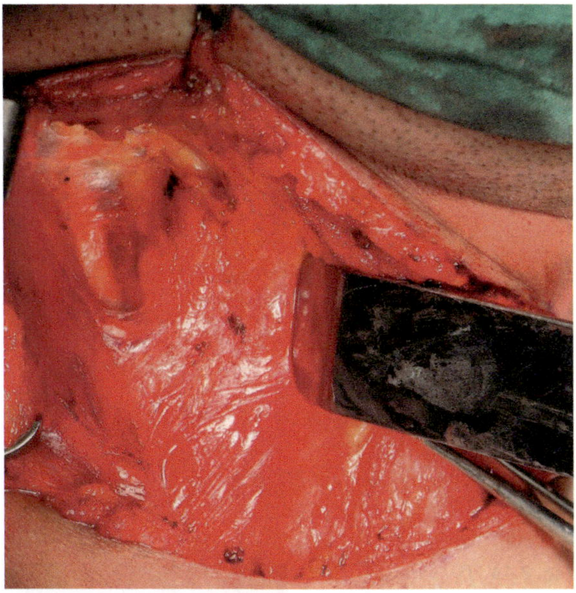

Fig. 8.11 IJV is exposed and anterior belly of digastric muscle seen

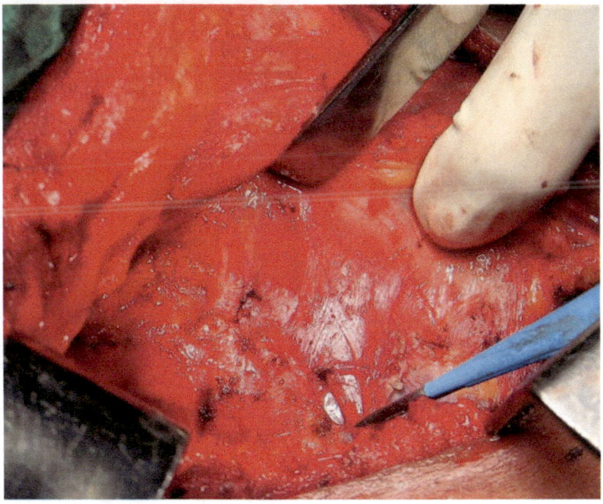

Fig. 8.12 Omohyoid muscle

medial sides of the IJV. The step is difficult when lymph nodes have peri-nodal infiltration and subsequent adhesion to the vessel. The mobilisation always starts at an area where the vessel is free (Fig. 8.15).

11. IJV is taped with vessel loops preferably at the middle portion. Adequate exposure with proper placements of retractors and focussing of light sources are essential. The first and second assistants are instructed to maintain steady but gentle retraction. A right-angle forceps is gently negotiated from the medial aspect to the lateral side lifting the vein exposing soft tissue. The vagus nerve is identified and safeguarded. The forceps is pushed further to open the avascular

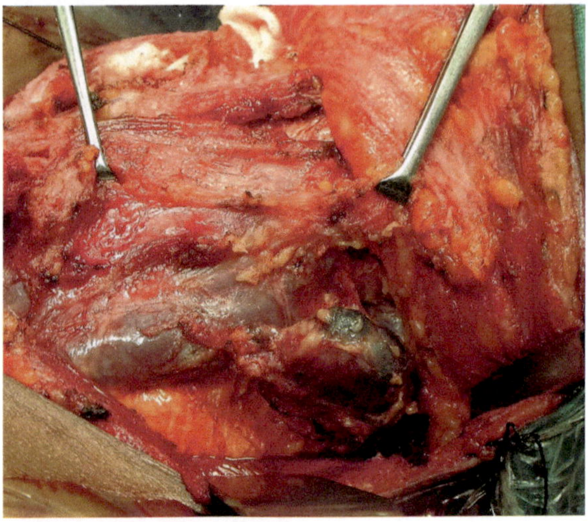

Fig. 8.13 Surface lymph nodes are dissected away

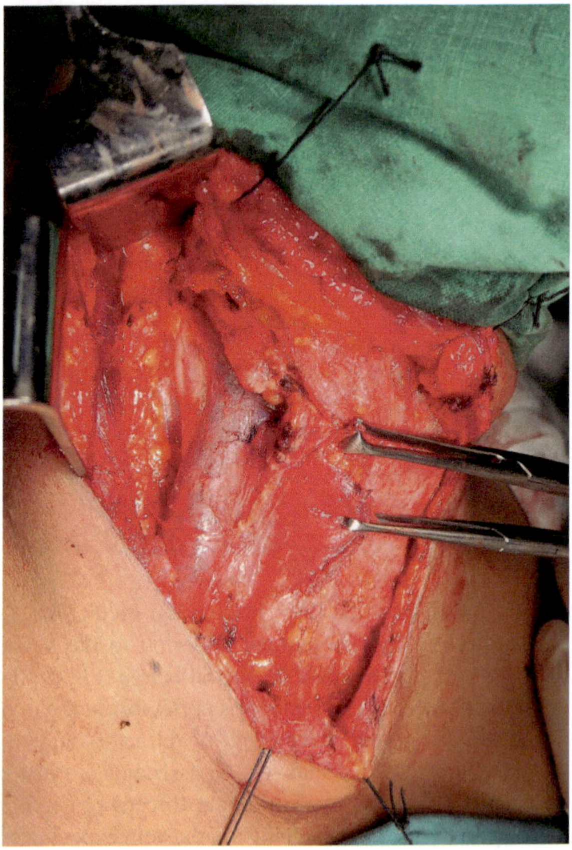

Fig. 8.14 IJV exposed

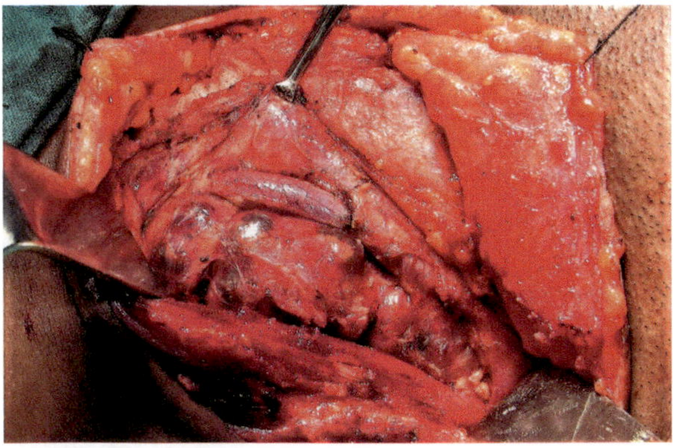

Fig. 8.15 Bulky nodes along lateral chain

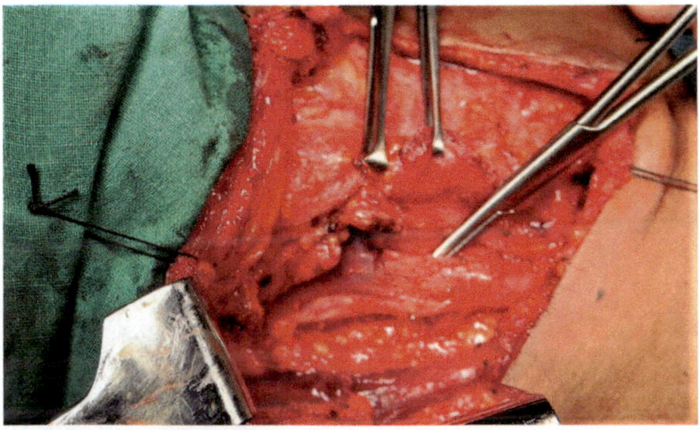

Fig. 8.16 Mobilization of IJV to pass a vessel tape

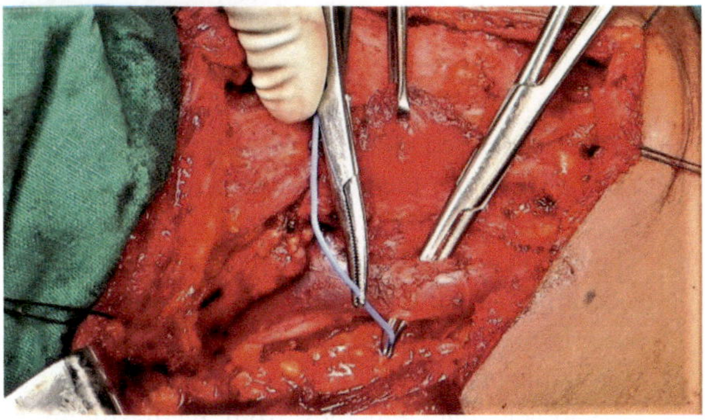

Fig. 8.17 Vessel loop taken around the IJV

soft tissue, then removed and reintroduced since a plug of soft tissue is usually adherent to the blade of forceps. The vessel loop is tucked and pulled up (Figs. 8.16, 8.17, and 8.18).

12. The lymph nodes are distributed posterior/lateral aspect of the vessel. The vein is held medially to expose the carotid vessel and vagus nerve. The surgeon stands on the side of the dissection from this step onwards. The first assistant holds the vessel loop and a vessel retractor to hold them medially. The SCM is

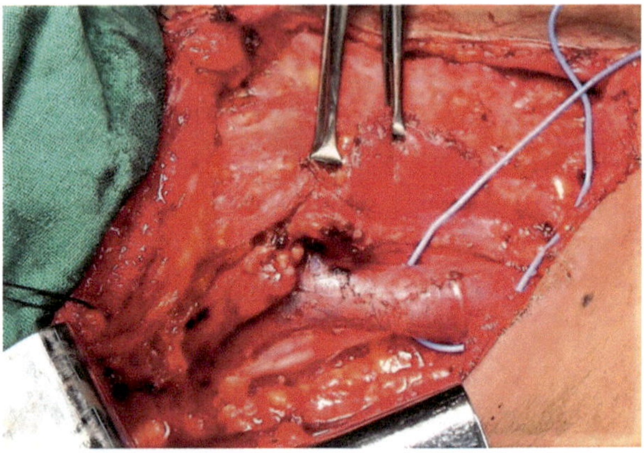

Fig. 8.18 Vagus seen behind the IJV

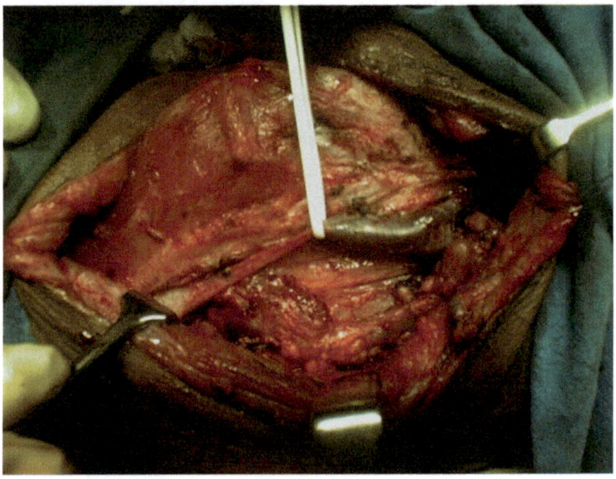

Fig. 8.19 Deep cervical lymph nodes exposed

further separated using a broad retractor or using tape encircled around the SCM. This tape facilitates lateral retraction of the SCM to expose Level V nodes also (Fig. 8.19).

13. The lymph node dissection starts from the lower part of the neck. IJV is retracted medially using the tape and a vein retractor may be used for additional exposure. Lymph nodes are seen posterior to IJV and removal of them is a crucial step in the procedure.

    Thoracic duct emerges from mediastinum on the left lateral aspect of oesophagus and courses deep to IJV and carotid artery to join the innominate vein. The duct loops in the neck and may extend as high as 4–6 cm before turning down to join the innominate vein. The thoracic duct has variable relation to IJV and hence careful and precise dissection is done in this area. The duct appears as a succulent near-transparent friable structure in the soft tissue. Lymph nodes of the region may empty directly to the duct and peri-nodal inflammatory changes are occasionally found. Lymph nodes in Level IV location may drain directly to the thoracic duct and any connections are better severed and ligated using 4-0 polypropylene sutures.

Injury thoracic duct is a rare complication of neck dissection and is better prevented than taking corrective measures. Thoracic duct injury is suspected when excess serous fluid accumulates in the lower aspect of the incision and chyle leak is not an intraoperative observation since the patient is starving for hours. After identifying the leak running sutures are applied using 4-0 polypropylene.

14. Phrenic nerve is deep to the scalene fascia and so can be easily safeguarded when perinodal adhesions are not present. If adhesions are noted lateral to medial dissection of nodal mass is done and the nerve is identified as it crosses the muscle deep to the fascia but clearly visible as a linear strand. The nodes posterior to the IJV at the lower part are removed under clear vision after identifying the thoracic duct and phrenic nerve. The phrenic nerve is safe so long as the scalene fascia is not breached (Figs. 8.20 and 8.21).

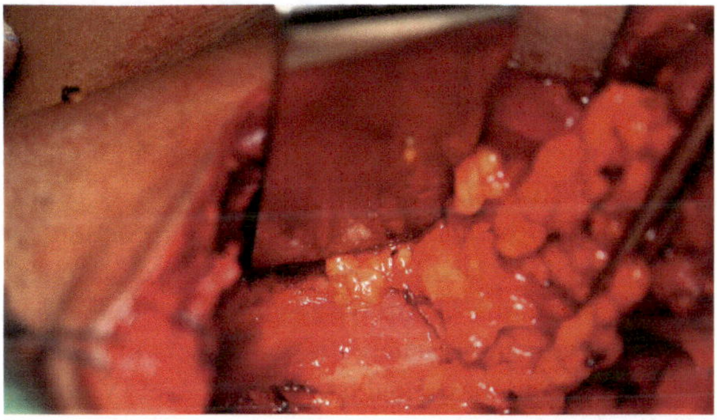

Fig. 8.20 Dissection of Level IV nodes exposing phrenic nerve

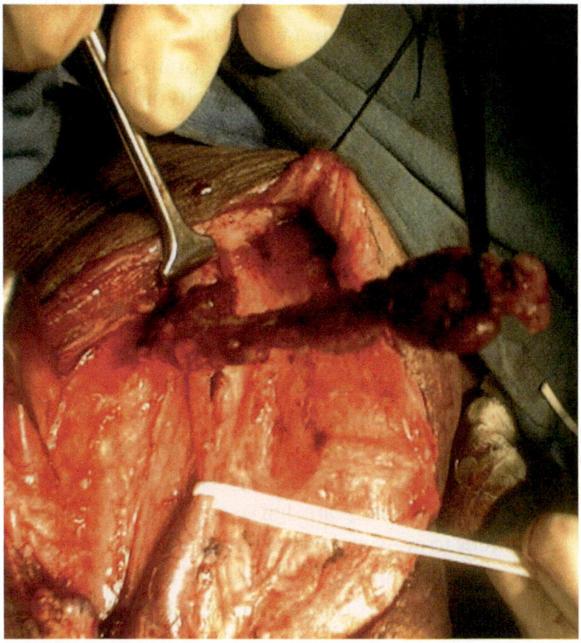

Fig. 8.21 Dissection of Level IV—lymph nodes completed

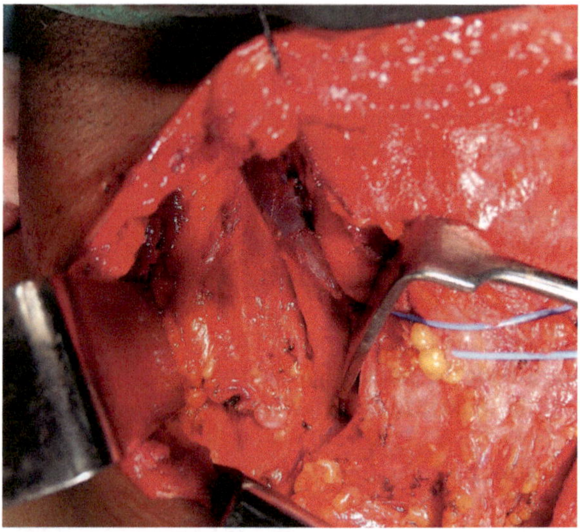

Fig. 8.22 Phrenic nerve and transverse cervical artery

15. Lymph nodes harvested from various stations are labelled separately for histological study. The transverse cervical artery is visualised and followed beyond the lateral border of the SCM and surrounding soft tissue and nodes are also removed and labelled separately as Level V nodes (Fig. 8.22).
16. The dissection of soft tissue superficial to the anterior scalene muscle is separated without breaching the deep fascia to the level of the cricoid cartilage and removed en-masse and labelled as Level IV nodes (Fig. 8.21).
17. Further dissection is continued towards the proximal part of IJV to the level of the hyoid bone. The spinal accessory nerve may be seen close to hyoid bone coursing to the medial border of SCM. But the venous tributaries are carefully controlled since they drain directly to IJV. The soft tissue with the lymph nodes to the level of the hyoid bone is removed and labelled as Level III (Fig. 8.23).
18. If dissection is to be extended to Level II area the spinal accessory is clearly defined from behind the posterior belly of the digastric muscle. The spinal accessory reaches the skull base jugular foramen and has variable relation to the IJV and reaches the posterior border of SCM. If lymph nodes are found close to SA nodes above and below are cleared taking extra care to the nerve (Fig. 8.24).
19. The first assistant shall steady the IJV and venous retractor for further exposure. A third assistant standing on the right side of the operator holds two deep-bladed Langenbeck retractors—one placed to retract the upper third of SCM and another to retract the posterior belly of the digastric muscle. The loop placed around the SCM may also be used for retraction.
20. The lymph nodes are harvested from this area with minimal use of energy sources to prevent thermal damage to the nerve. Careful haemostasis is achieved by judicious use of haemostatic clips. The soft tissue with lymph nodes is labelled as Level IIa and IIb accordingly (Figs. 8.24 and 8.25).

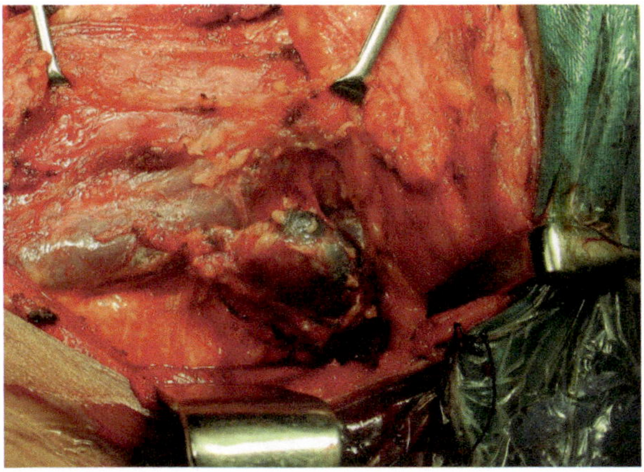

Fig. 8.23 Level III nodes

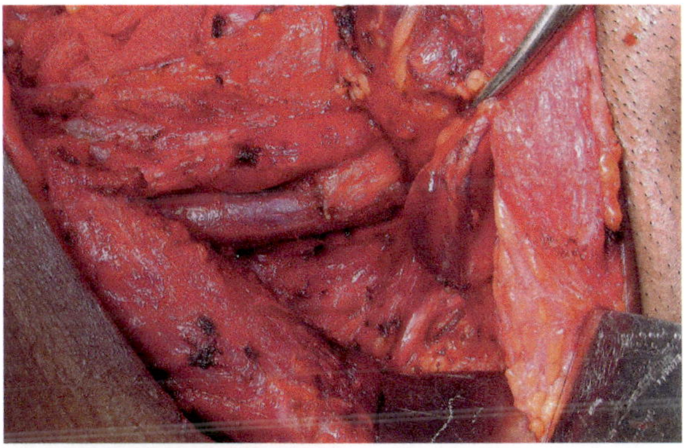

Fig. 8.24 Level II nodes

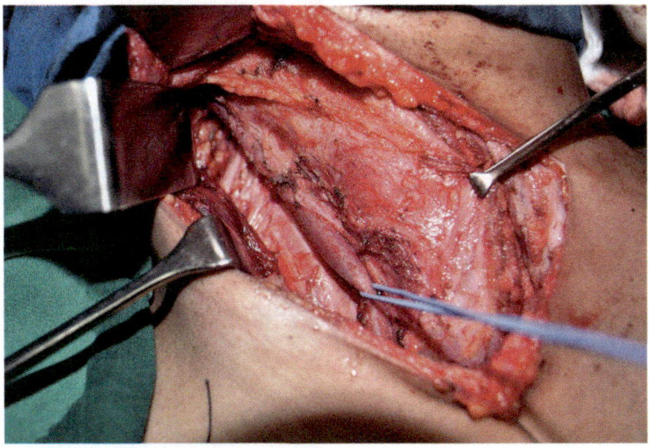

Fig. 8.25 Dissection of Level IIa and IIb completed

21. Haemostasis is ensured. The area of the thoracic duct is inspected for accumulation of fluid. If suspected of injury careful examination of the area and identify the site of the leak. The duct is ligated using 4-0 polypropylene sutures (Figs. 8.26, 8.27, and 8.28).

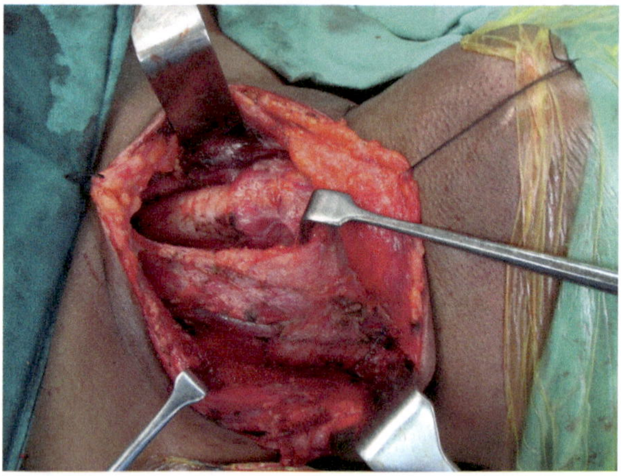

Fig. 8.26 Inspection of field after TT + MRND

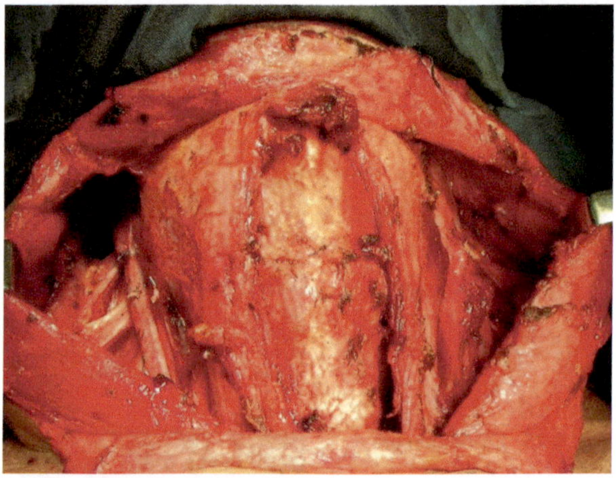

Fig. 8.27 Inspection of surgical site after completion of procedure—bilateral dissection

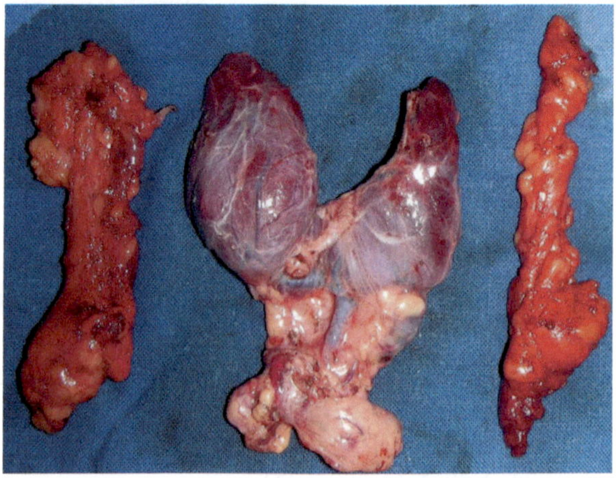

Fig. 8.28 Total thyroidectomy, central compartment dissection and bilateral neck dissection—specimen

22. A 12 F suction drain is inserted through a stab incision close to the lateral end of the skin incision. Investing layer of deep fascia is sutured using 3-0 polyglactin sutures and skin closed subcuticular continuous suture using 4-0 Poliglecaprone. An occlusive dressing is kept covering the incision.

8.3 Postoperative Care

The patient is observed in the postoperative care room for 6 h and systematically ambulated. Generally, prophylaxis for venous thrombosis is not necessary since early ambulation is possible. Routine perioperative or prophylactic antibiotic therapy is not indicated.

The suction drain is maintained for 24–48 h and removed. The majority of patients are discharged after 48 h.

Complications: Reactionary haemorrhage is an occasional complication and can be disastrous. Since they are draining directly to the internal jugular massive bleeding may occur and is usually found during the early hours after the operation. The haematoma tracks to the central compartment and causes dyspnoea due to laryngeal oedema.

The accessory nerve is a composite nerve having a cranial root and cervical root. The cranial portion joins the vagus nerve and the spinal portion innervates sterno-cleido-mastoid (SCM) and trapezius muscles. The common trunk after exiting from the brain through the jugular foramen bifurcates to the cranial portion which joins the vagus and spinal portion which progresses to the under the surface of the upper portion of SCM. The nerve enters SCM approximately 5 cm inferior to the apex of the mastoid and leaves it posteriorly at the level of the superior border of the thyroid cartilage. The nerve exits from the SCM along the posterior border and courses trapezius just deep to the deep fascia. Iatrogenic injury to the accessory nerve is frequent when dissecting posterior triangle to remove Level V nodes a nodal station that is rarely approached in segment-oriented dissection for thyroid cancers. But the trunk of the nerve during its course towards SCM is at risk during Level II dissection. Most of the accessory nerve injuries are due to traction or thermal injury from the lateral spread of energy sources. The characteristic shoulder pain and disability in movements are called shoulder syndrome. Failure to recognise the condition sufficiently early leads to a permanent disability of the shoulder. The basic principle is early detection and adopting measures to retain functionally active trapezius muscle.

Physical therapy to maintain trapezius function and periodic reviews to assess the progress is initiated as early as possible. Nonsteroidal anti-inflammatory drugs and transcutaneous nerve stimulation are complementary to routine physical therapy. The majority of patients recover completely since transactions are rare.

Thoracic duct injury is a rare complication of thyroidectomies and cervical block dissections amounting to 0.5–8%. The thoracic duct reaches a recess on the root of the neck bounded medially by the oesophagus, laterally by omohyoid muscle, posteriorly by vertebra, and anteriorly by the carotid sheath. Generally, 3–5 cm cervical course of the thoracic duct is over the anterior scalene muscle and enters the innominate vein near the confluence. Rarely cervical course may be longer and higher reaching even up to the hyoid bone. The thoracic duct empties lymph whole left side and part of the right-side body which includes the intestine also. The thoracic duct is at risk when Level IV nodes close to the confluence are dissected and also in central compartment dissection reaching close to the innominate vein.

During the surgical procedure, thoracic duct injury is suspected when the excessive discharge of any nature wells up the surgical wound. The accumulating fluid may not have classical nature of chyle since the patients are starving. Identification of thoracic duct may require magnification and the injured duct is ligated with nonabsorbable material. Placement of ligature is tricky since the duct is easily friable. A muscle flap from the clavicular head of SCM or anterior scalene is used for reinforcement [1].

Chyle leaks manifest during the immediate postoperative period as excessive drainage and used to have the typical appearance of chyle. Chyle leak is almost always diagnosed clinically by the nature of fluid but the presence of high triglyceride (>100 mg/dL) and chylomicrons confirms the diagnosis. The leak is considered high output when it is >500 mL/24 h and a low output when it is less than 500 mL/24 h.

Low output chyle leak is managed conservatively and with restriction of physical activities, and dietary regulations. Physical activity increases chyle flow low fat diet or non-fat diet is preferable to reduce chyle. Recovery of low output fistula occurs early but high output fistula may be refractory to these measures alone. If the output does not significantly reduce in 48 h aggressive management with oral intake is restricted total parenteral nutrition may be initiated.

In refractory patients, somatostatin or its long-acting analogue, octreotide is found highly useful. Octreotide in doses ranging from 100 to 200 μg administered subcutaneously for 7 days controls chyle leak effectively in the majority of cases.

Re-surgery is required in selected patients when all other measures are exhausted suture closure over muscle flap is attempted. Compression dressings are generally applied but have a questionable effect.

Phrenic nerve injury is a very rare complication of MRND. The phrenic nerve supplies motor innervation to the diaphragm which is of paramount importance in respiration. The nerve courses deep to scalene fascia and is at risk when dissecting lymph nodes with perinodal infiltration. The unilateral phrenic nerve palsy may pass unnoticed in a few patients or with minimal symptoms as dyspnoea on exertion. Bilateral paralysis is always very symptomatic and disabling the patient. Ultrasound imaging diaphragm appears as an echogenic line with a thickness of 22–28 mm. Thinning of the muscle mass of the diaphragm and paradoxical movements are diagnostic of paralysis. Of the various treatment options plication of the muscle of the affected side is found very useful.

Reference

1. Delaney SW, Shi H, Shokrani A, Sinha UK. Management of chyle leak after head and neck surgery: review current treatment strategies. Int J Otolaryngol. 2017;2017:8362874.

Trans-oral Endoscopic Thyroidectomy via Vestibular Approach (TOETVA)

9

Gyan Chand

9.1 Introduction

The conventional open surgical procedures for thyroid and parathyroid diseases result in scars on the front of the neck and are cosmetically unacceptable for many patients. The remote access thyroid and parathyroid surgical procedures were first introduced in 1996 [1, 2], and there was considerable interest among patients and surgeons. Subsequently, many innovations in surgical techniques and instruments were introduced. Newer energy sources for haemostasis, neuromonitoring systems, and surgical robots improved the outcomes of remote access procedures. The remote access procedures shifted the incisions to relatively hidden regions resulting in extensive dissections. The trans-oral approach shifts the scar to the natural orifice.

Witzel et al.'s pioneering efforts in 2008 paved the way for Trans-oral Endoscopic Thyroid Surgery (TOETS) [1]. They removed the thyroid first in human cadavers and later in live pigs through the trans-oral approach. Wilhelm and Metzig introduced a change in approach through sublingual and vestibular locations. Modifications to this natural orifice approach in thyroid surgery were reported by various authors, including the lateral sublingual approach by Karakas et al. [3], and Nakajo et al.'s vestibular approach complemented with a mechanical retracting system [4]. A tri-vestibular approach was proposed by Wang et al. [5] and Anuwong [6] for thyroidectomy aided by a constant gas insufflation. A robotic arm was used by Lee et al. [7], but an additional port in the contralateral axilla was also used.

The trans-oral vestibular approach to the thyroid gland is the shortest midline approach with minimal dissection. Since it is through a natural orifice there is no visible scar and ensuring excellent cosmesis. This chapter describes the technique of endoscopic trans-oral thyroidectomy via the vestibular approach, emphasising the selection of patients and surgical technique.

G. Chand (✉)
Endocrine Surgery, SGPGI, Lucknow, Uttar Pradesh, India

C. G. Nair, S. J. Abraham (eds.), *Surgical Management of Thyroid and Parathyroid Diseases*, https://doi.org/10.1007/978-981-97-3774-1_9

Table 9.1 Selection criteria for TOETVA

Indications	Contraindications
Thyroid diameter <10 cm and dominant nodule <6 cm (Bethesda II, III or IV lesions)	Previous head and neck surgery or radiation at neck and upper mediastinum
Thyroid nodule <2 cm when the cytology shows Bethesda V or VI	Lymph node metastasis or locally advanced thyroid cancer
Selected Grave's disease	Uncontrolled toxic goitres or sub-sternal thyroidal extension
History of scar hypertrophy	Patient unfit for surgery or general anaesthesia
Motivated patient to avoid a cervical neck incision	Preoperative RLN palsy or oral abscess

9.2 Indications of TOETVA

The careful selection of the patient plays a vital role in the success of the endoscopic trans-oral thyroidectomy via the vestibular approach. Patient features such as age, body habitus, and personal preference to avoid a neck scar are essential prerequisites. Generally, nontoxic nodules less than 30 mm in size are considered ideal for trans-oral procedures. The procedure may be offered for nodular goitre, papillary microcarcinoma and Graves' disease.

Early in the beginning Anuwong et al. and Jitpratoom et al. recommended a maximum allowable nodule diameter of 10 cm, while Wang et al. suggested an 8 cm maximum size. But recently the suggested maximum diameter of nodules ranged from 4 to 6 cm (Kim et al.; Richmond et al.) [8–10].

The current indications and contraindications for the selection of patients for endoscopic thyroid surgery via vestibular approach (TOETVA) are listed in Table 9.1.

9.3 Preoperative Evaluation

The preoperative investigations and preparations are not different. When the cytology suggests malignancy, a neck and upper mediastinum CT scan is done. The thyroid dysfunction is corrected, and the patient is rendered euthyroid.

Proper preoperative counselling, narrating the details of the procedure, determining the chances of complications and onverting to an open procedure in any adverse situation, are of paramount significance. Detailed informed consent is always recorded.

Proper oral hygiene is always ensured, and chlorhexidine mouthwashes are given for two weeks before the planned operation. Clipping of hair from neck, axilla and chest wall is done.

9.4 Surgical Technique of TOETVA

- **Anaesthesia and Position**
  - General anaesthesia with nasal endotracheal intubation is routine, and the tube is fixed to the forehead with a pad support. A suitable eye ointment is applied, and eyes are covered with a waterproof covering like Ioban™ drapes.
  - The patient is supine with the neck extended, keeping a roll under the shoulder and both arms adducted at the shoulder joint. The monitors and anaesthesia machines are moved to the foot end.
  - Antiseptic painting is done on the lower face, neck, and upper chest with iodine solution. The oral cavity is cleansed twice with chlorhexidine mouthwash, and the throat is packed with ribbon gauge. Sterile drapes were placed and marked the anatomical landmarks, including thyroid cartilage, sternal notch, and medial border of the bilateral sternocleidomastoid muscle (SCM), with skin markers
  - Perioperative antibiotic is given just before placing the incision
- **Instruments**
  - The conventional general laparoscopic set, along with the required energy devices
  - 5 or 10-mm endoscope (0 and 30°)
  - Three ports (one 10 mm central and two 5 mm lateral)
  - Laparoscopic alligator forceps
  - Laparoscopic Maryland dissector
  - Laparoscopic mini hook cautery
  - Laparoscopic needle holder
  - 5 mm laparoscopic ultrasonic scalpel
  - 5 mm endoscopic suction irrigation
  - Endoscopic peanut
- **Procedure**
  - Step 1

    A central horizontal incision of 10 mm is done through the vestibular mucosa and submucosa of the lower lip to reach the periosteum of the mandible. Dilute adrenaline solution (1:200 by volume) is injected in the midline with a Veress needle in the sub-platysmal plane of the marked area in the neck. A blind dissection is done in the subplatysmal plane over the neck with a vascular tunneler or a custom-made tunneler and used to wait for 2 min to ensure haemostasis.

Two 5 mm vertical incisions were made in the vestibular mucosa of the lower lip at the level of both canine teeth.

- Step 2

  A 10 mm trocar is inserted and connected with a CO2 insufflator and pressure is maintained at a 6–7 mmHg. The lower part of neck is compressed to prevent emphysema or air embolism.

  Diluted adrenaline saline solution is infiltrated at lateral 5 mm incisions, and 5 mm trocars are introduced.

- Step 3

  The camera and energy devise are now introduced, and dissection is continued under vision in the subplatysmal plane. A flap is raised in this plane, extending laterally up to the sides of the sternomastoid and inferiorly to the suprasternal notch.

  The hook cautery is now used to open the midline avascular facia between the strap muscles. The retraction of strap muscles exposes the isthmus of the thyroid.

  The alligator forceps is used to hold the isthmus and pulled to opposite side of dissection. The strap muscle is separated from lateral aspect of the lobe using harmonic scalpel.

  A suture is negotiated from outside at the level of the cricoid cartilage encircling the SCM and returns back outside the skin to retract the SCM.

  The lateral dissection is continued to identify the superior parathyroid and then dissection is directed caudally towards the lower pole.

  Lateral thyroid dissection should be done carefully, and if the middle thyroid vein is encountered, coagulate and divide with the energy device. The Reeve's or cricothyroid space is opened, and the superior thyroid vessels are exposed clearly. The external division of the superior laryngeal nerve is now identified before dividing the superior thyroid vessels with energy sources.

  After the superior thyroid vessels are securely divided, the pole is rotated medially, and the dissection is continued to identify the superior parathyroid and recurrent laryngeal nerve. The tubercle of Zuckerkandl is an excellent landmark for identifying the recurrent laryngeal nerve. When facilities are available for neuro-monitoring, the RLN is easily identified, especially in the presence of adhesions and enlarged lymph nodes.

The nerve is followed the entire length, and its relation to the inferior thyroid artery and thyroid is noted before the removal of the gland starts. The tiny blood vessels crossing the nerve are secured using Ligaclips.

After separating the RLN, the thyroid lobe is dissected from the trachea.

The inferior parathyroid gland is visualised and preserved. The inferior thyroid veins are divided, and the lower pole is freed from the soft tissue.

- Step 4

  The lobe is entirely separated from the trachea using energy sources placed in an endo-bag and removed through the central vestibular incision. In the case of a large specimen, the lobe is divided into smaller pieces and removed or may be extracted through the axilla by an additional port.

  A similar procedure is continued on the other side for a total thyroidectomy.

  A perfect haemostasis is ensured before the midline is sutured with 3-0 Polyglactin (vicryl) sutures after applying the haemostatic agent in the thyroid bed.

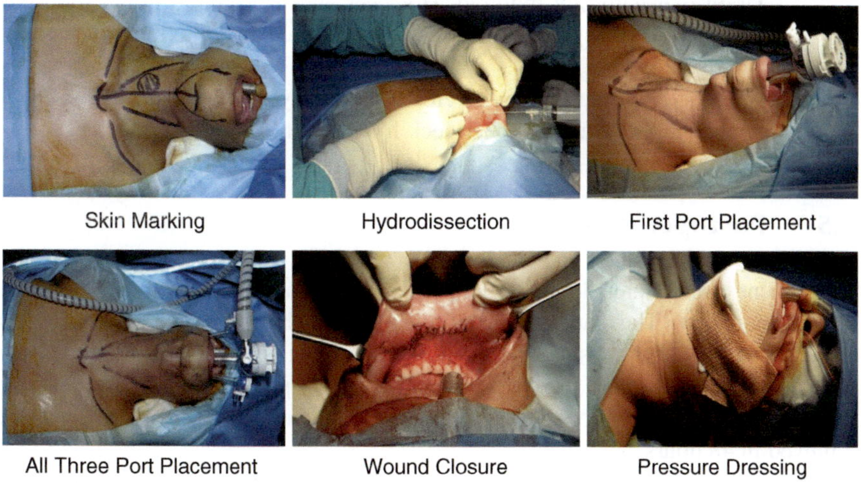

Fig. 9.1 The technical aspect of endoscopic thyroid surgery via trans-oral vestibular approach

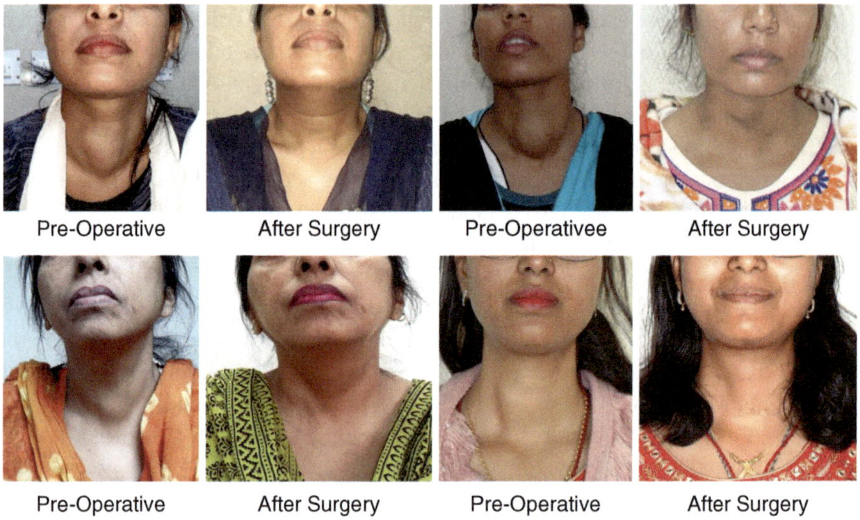

Fig. 9.2 Cosmetic outcome of endoscopic thyroid surgery via trans-oral vestibular approach

Drain is usually not required. However, when placing a drain, the tip is brought out through the posterior aspect of the neck or axilla.

– Step 5

The vestibular incisions were closed in two layers, the pressure dressing is applied at the chin and upper neck for 12–24 h (Figs. 9.1 and 9.2).

9.5 Postoperative Care

The patient is ambulated 4 hours after surgery, and oral fluids usually start 6 hours after the surgery. The patient is continued on prophylactic oral antibiotics for 5–7 days. All patients are suggested to perfect oral hygiene by using mouth washes after every meal for Seven days. Postoperative care of patients is not different from those undergone conventional open thyroidectomy. The drain, when kept, shall be removed in 48 hours.

The majority of patients are discharged within 24 h following a hemithyroidectomy. Patients are discharged on the 4th or 5th day following total thyroidectomy.

Patients are systematically observed for hypocalcaemia, and management of hypocalcaemia is not different.

9.6 Outcome

Trans-oral thyroid surgery is being practised by several surgeons in hospitals worldwide. They perform all forms of thyroid surgery successfully, including lobectomies, hemithyroidectomies, total thyroidectomies, etc., in various pathological indications like benign symptomatic to asymptomatic malignancies. A proper preoperative assessment and selection of patients avoid the possibility of conversion to an open procedure. The postoperative hospital stay is very variable, depending on the extent of surgery and thyroid pathology.

The usual complications, including hypoparathyroidism, recurrent laryngeal nerve injury, postoperative hematoma, and surgical site infection, are similar to conventional open thyroid surgery. Some specific complications include skin burns, mental nerve injury, and paraesthesia over the chin and upper part of the neck, which is managed conservatively.

9.7 Operative Safety

Trans-oral thyroid surgery is no longer considered a novel technique or experimental technique. Several studies have been published around the world, revealing the safety and efficacy of this technique; however, no specific guideline has been established to consider who is capable of performing endoscopic trans-oral surgery. The experts suggest that the surgeon should have expertise in thyroid surgery and be well-experienced in endoscopic surgery. The learning curve guideline is also not mentioned; however, the expert found that more than 15 independent surgeries under expert guidance are sufficient to develop true proficiency in this procedure.

9.8 Conclusion

The endoscopic trans-oral thyroid surgery via vestibular approach is a technically feasible, safe, midline approach with minimal invasion for benign and malignant thyroid excision, providing excellent cosmetic outcomes.

References

1. Gagner M. Endoscopic subtotal parathyroidectomy in patients with primary hyperparathyroidism. Br J Surg. 1996;83(6):875.
2. Hüscher CS, Chiodini S, Napolitano C, Recher A. Endoscopic right thyroid lobectomy. Surg Endosc. 1997;11(8):877.
3. Wong KP, Lang Brian HH. Endoscopic thyroidectomy: a literature review and update. Curr Surg Rep. 2013;1:7–15.
4. Gagner M, Inabent BW III, Biertho L. Endoscopic thyroidectomy for solitary nodules. Ann Chir. 2013;128:696–701.
5. Cougard P, Osmak L, Esquis P, Ognois P. Endoscopic thyroidectomy: a preliminary report including 40 patients. Ann Chir. 2005;130:81–5.
6. Inabent WB III, Jacob BP, Gagner M. Minimally invasive endoscopic thyroidectomy by cervical approach. Surg Endosc. 2003;17:1808–11.
7. Henry JF, Sebag F. Lateral endoscopic approach for thyroid and parathyroid surgery. Ann Chir. 2006;131:51–6.

8. Choo JM, You JY, Kim HY, Overview and suggestions for future research in new minimally invasive thyroid surgery. J Minim Invasive Surg. 2019;22(1):5–10. https://doi.org/10.7602/jmis.2019.22.1.5.
9. Richmon JD, Kim HY. Transoral robotic thyroidectomy (TORT): procedures and outcomes. Gland Surg. 2017;6(3):285–9. https://doi.org/10.21037/gs.2017.05.05.
10. Anuwong A. Transoral endoscopic thyroidectomy vestibular approach: a series of the first 60n human cases. World J Surg. 2016;40(3):491–7.

Robotic Thyroidectomy

10

Krishnakumar Thankappan, Nisha Rajrattansingh Akali, Nageswara Rao Noothanapati, Snigdha Elaprolu, and Lakshmi Ravunniarth Menon

10.1 Introduction

The Framingham study in 1968 demonstrated an overall prevalence of thyroid nodules in the general population of 4.2% [1]. It is a common endocrine disorder, more so in females. Incidental thyroid nodules that are detected in an imaging study performed for other reasons is a common scenario. Hepatobiliary and gastrointestinal surgeons routinely perform minimally invasive and remote access procedures. Such a procedure aims to reduce postoperative morbidity, pain, promote decreased hospital stay, and provide cosmesis.

Endoscopic thyroidectomy was first performed in 1997 [2]. Since then, various remote access methods have been introduced via the axilla, breast, anterior chest, and post-auricular route. However, the endoscopic route is met with limitations of narrow working space, two-dimensional view, and a restricted area of instrument manipulation. An assistant is required to hold the camera.

Robotic-assisted thyroid surgery (RATS) is gaining popularity because of its promise of being a scarless (in the neck) procedure. This a quite an attractive option especially in young women and in cultural communities where a horizontal neck scar can have different perceptions. The da Vinci robotic system (Intuitive Surgical, Sunnyvale, California) was first utilised for trans-axillary thyroidectomy by Chung in 2007 [3]. Since then, there has been a rapid increase in cases of robotic thyroidectomy done mainly in South Korea.

K. Thankappan (✉) · N. R. Akali · N. R. Noothanapati · S. Elaprolu · L. R. Menon
Department of Head and Neck Surgery, Amrita Institute of Medical Sciences, Amrita Vishwa Vidyapeetham, Kochi, Kerala, India

C. G. Nair, S. J. Abraham (eds.), *Surgical Management of Thyroid and Parathyroid Diseases*, https://doi.org/10.1007/978-981-97-3774-1_10

10.2 Evolution of Minimal Invasive and Remote Access Surgical Approaches to the Thyroid

First endoscopic subtotal parathyroidectomy was described in the literature by Cleveland general surgeon, M. Gagner, in 1995, using 5 mm 30° endoscope and carbon-di-oxide insufflation. But, the patient developed hypercarbia and extensive subcutaneous emphysema (from eyes to scrotum), which were managed conservatively [4]. The endoscopic approach for thyroid tumour was first described by Italian general surgeons using an endoscope, wall lifter and low-pressure CO_2 insufflation. They found that the wall lifter with low CO_2 insufflation limited the effects of hypercarbia and subcutaneous emphysema [2]. Miccoli and colleagues pioneered the minimally invasive video-assisted thyroidectomy (MIVAT) and assured the safety of the procedure in both benign and malignant small thyroid nodules on a large scale (336 patients) with multi-institutional experience (Italy, Belgium and Germany) [5].

Japanese surgeons, Ohgami et al. (2000), published their experience of feasibility and safety of endoscopic thyroidectomy using the breast approach with 15 mm incision between the nipples and CO_2 insufflation (6 mmHg), and named this procedure as "Scarless endoscopic thyroidectomy" [6]. Another Japanese team, Ikeda et al. demonstrated endoscopic thyroidectomy by the axillary approach using a 30 mm skin incision and CO_2 insufflation (4 mmHg), where the small scar is completely hidden in the axilla [7]. Various modifications are described in the literature by multiple authors in the endoscopic breast and axillary approach [8–10]. Korean group Lee et al. demonstrated the postauricular and axillary approach endoscopic neck surgery for thyroidectomy with 12 mm axillary incision, postauricular ports and CO_2 insufflation (5–6 mmHg) [11]. Thomas Wilhelm (German ENT surgeon) et al. demonstrated a combined sublingual and bi-vestibular trans-oral endoscopic approach for thyroid on cadavers based on the natural orifice surgery (NOS) principle [12]. Same approach was applied on a 53-year-old male patient for thyroidectomy with 5 mm sub-lingual incision and CO_2 insufflation (6 mmHg) [13]. Several modifications were described in literature based on NOS principle such as gasless premandible trans-oral video-assisted neck surgery (TOVANS) [14], trans-oral vestibular approach on cadavers [15], and modified trans-vestibular approach first on cadavers followed by clinically on 30 years old female [16, 17].

Robotic surgery eliminates the limitations of endoscopic surgery, such as gas inflation was replaced by using the retractors, three-dimensional view (3D vision), and "wristed instruments" with 7° of freedom and elimination of hand tremors. Korean surgical team was the first to apply robotic technology in thyroid surgery by gasless trans-axillary approach for thyroid cancer [18]. This team used the da Vinci S surgical robot system on 100 patients without any serious complications. Walvekar et al. described the retro auricular video-assisted "gas-less" thyroidectomy on human cadavers and also mentioned the value of incorporating robotic technology in this approach [19]. Georgia-based ENT surgeons Terris and Singer described the novel technique of retro auricular robotic facelift thyroidectomy without any complications and drain on an outpatient basis [20]. Korea-based surgeons, Lee et al. described the trans-oral robotic thyroidectomy first on live porcine models and human cadavers followed by on live patients without any complications and difficulty except temporary mental nerve paraesthesia in three cases [21]. Table 10.1 shows a classification of minimally invasive and remote access approaches to the thyroid. Table 10.2 shows a comparison of open, endoscopic and robotic thyroidectomy.

Table 10.1 Classification of surgical approaches. Minimally invasive and remote access surgical approaches to the thyroid divided into direct approaches (cervical) and indirect approaches (extra-cervical)

Surgical approach	Type of approach	Incisions/ports
Direct/cervical approaches	Video assisted central approach, gasless or MIVAT	
	Lateral endoscopic approach	Single incision Multiple incision
	Anterior endoscopic approach	Single incision Multiple incision
Indirect/extra-cervical/ remote access approaches (both endoscopic and robotic)	Trans-axillary approach	
	Breast approach	ABBA BABA
	Chest wall approach	
	Retro-auricular approach	
	Trasoral approach or NOS approach (natural orifice surgery)	
	TARA approach (trans-axillary and retro-auricular)	

Table 10.2 A comparison of open, endoscopic and robotic thyroidectomy

Variable	Open thyroidectomy	Endoscopic thyroidectomy	Robotic thyroidectomy
Scar	Visible	Negligible	Hidden
Operating time	Less	More	More
Dissection	Standard	More extensive	More extensive but precise, dexterity
Visualization	Naked eye	2-dimensional	3-dimensional
Pain	Minimal	More, in the chest wall	More, in the chest wall/ neck
Recurrent laryngeal nerve palsy	Similar	Similar	Similar
Hypocalcemia	Similar	Similar	Similar
Cosmesis	Visible scar	Better	Better
Oncologic outcomes	Good and proven	Less data	Less data, can do neck dissection
Cost	Standard	Costlier	Two to eight times than endoscopic
Learning curve	Standard	More	Less than endoscopic

10.3 Indications

Young women or patients who want to avoid a neck scar, patients with a history of hypertrophic scars or keloid are the ideal candidates for RATS. However, better cosmesis is not the only reason. Robotic surgery has its own added advantages. The thyroid pathology will influence selecting the approach. The presence of thyroiditis is a relative contraindication due to associated fibrosis and adhesions. Malignancy as such is not a contraindication [22]. Ideal patients include:

- Small or average-sized (BMI <30) young patients
- Concerns of neck scarring, or history of keloid or hypertrophic scar
- An indeterminate thyroid lesion less than 4 cm in diameter or confirmed papillary thyroid cancers less than 3 cm in diameter
- Multinodular goitres with smaller (<4 cm) nodules
- Total thyroid volume <40 mL

10.4 Contraindications

The contraindications may be relative or absolute [22].

10.4.1 Relative

1. Well-differentiated thyroid cancers >T2
2. Thyroid nodules >4 cm
3. Larger goitres (thyroid volume >40 mL)
4. Severe Grave's disease with enlarged glands
5. Advanced thyroiditis

10.4.2 Absolute

1. Thyroid cancer with evidence of gross invasion
2. Previous neck surgery or irradiation
3. A substernal or retrosternal goitre
4. Morbid obesity

The American Thyroid Association has published a statement indicating that remote-access thyroidectomy may be performed safely in high volume areas in selected patients and strict selection criteria [23].

10.5 Surgical Techniques of Robotic Thyroidectomy

10.5.1 Retro-auricular approach—Robotic thyroidectomy

The technique followed by the authors' group has been reported in a separate article [24]. The equipment and the steps of the procedure are summarised below.

10.5.1.1 Surgical Equipment

Skin flap retractors

- Skin hooks
- Army navy retractors
- Langenbach's retractors of different sizes
- Self-retaining retractor (L&C Bio Co, South Korea) (Fig. 10.1a, b)

Instruments for gross dissection

- Monopolar cautery with tips of three different sizes: small, medium, and long
- Debakey forceps
- Yankauer suction tips (plastic and longer metal type)

Surgical robot

The authors use the da Vinci Xi system (Intuitive Surgical Systems, Sunnyvale, CA, USA). Si version is also available. The operation room scene is depicted in Fig. 10.2. Three components of the system are (1) the patient cart, (2) the vision cart, and (3) the surgeon console (Fig. 10.3a–c). The instruments used have minor variations depending on the model used.

For Si model

- 12 mm, 30° facedown endoscope
- 5-mm Maryland forceps
- 5-mm harmonic curved scissors
- 5-mm monopolar cautery
- 8-mm Prograsp forceps

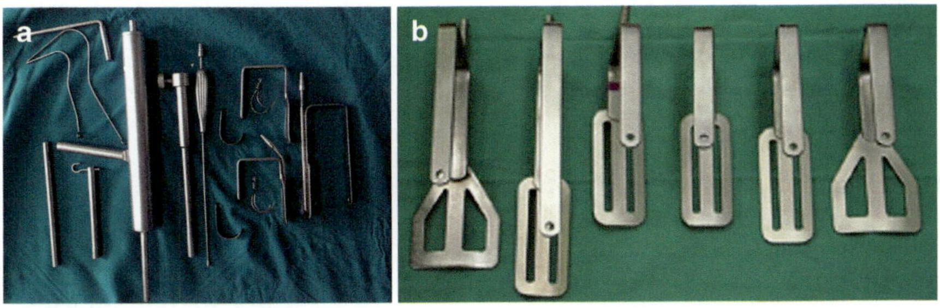

Fig. 10.1 (**a**, **b**) Self retaining retractors for retro-auricular robotic thyroidectomy

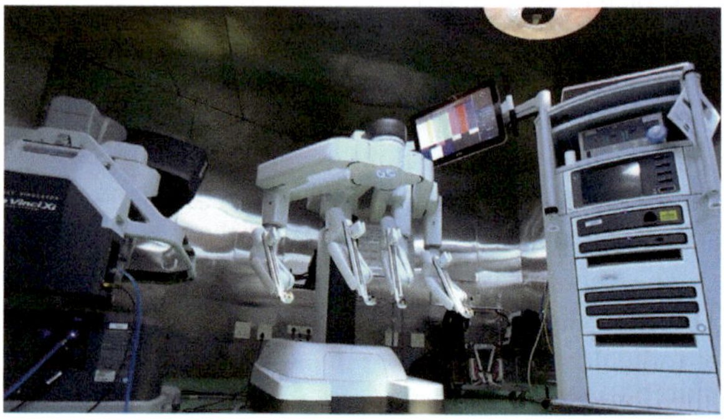

Fig. 10.2 Operating room for robotic thyroidectomy

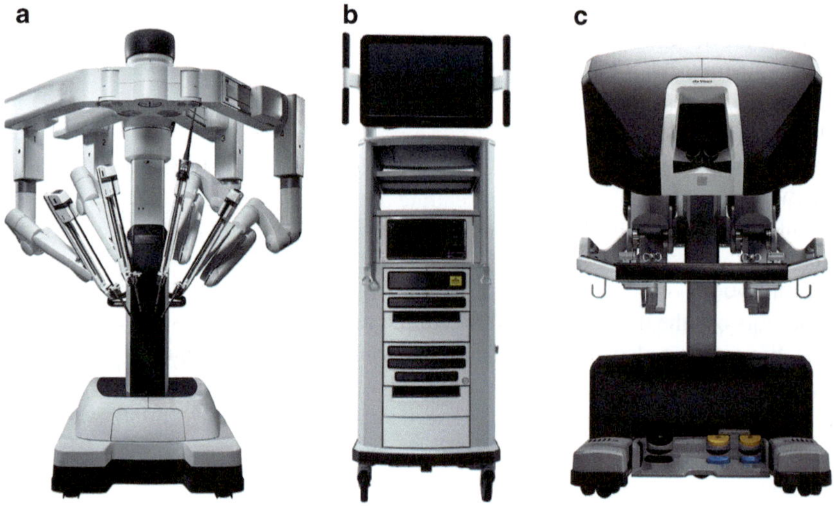

Fig. 10.3 (**a**) Patient console, da Vinci robotic system; (**b**) Vision cart, da Vinci robotic system; (**c**) Surgeon console, da Vinci robotic system

For Xi model

- 8-mm 30° facedown endoscope
- 8-mm bipolar Maryland forceps
- 8-mm monopolar curved scissors
- 8-mm monopolar spatula tip
- 8-mm Prograsp forceps

Vessel ligation clip system

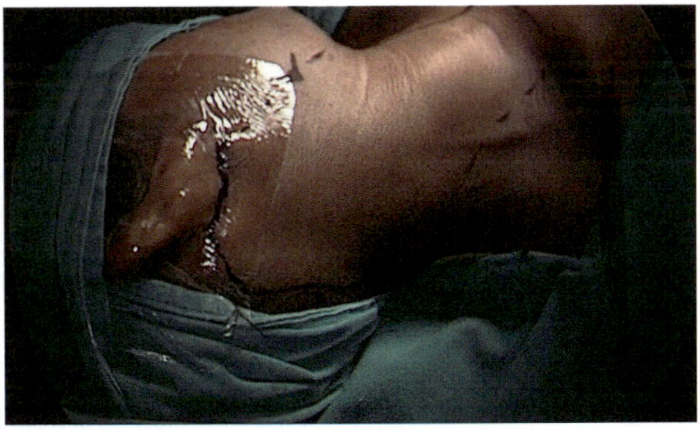

Fig. 10.4 Retro-auricular incision

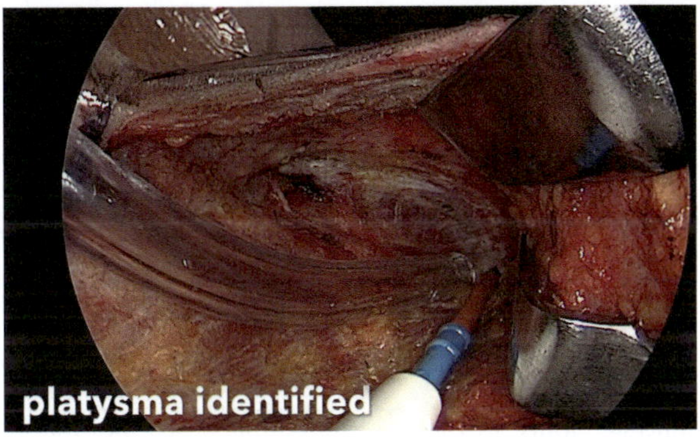

Fig. 10.5 Retro-auricular, working space being created

10.5.1.2 Preparation and Procedure

Patient Positioning

The patient is placed in the supine position with the head rotated to the contralateral side. The neck is placed in the natural position. No extension is required. Ipsilateral ear lobule can be folded away with a Tegaderm dressing.

Skin Preparation and Incision

Retro-auricular incision (Fig. 10.4) is marked along the occipital hairline then joins the postauricular crease avoiding the acute angle. The marked area can be infiltrated with vasoconstrictors to maintain a bloodless field. The working corridor can also be marked to limit to avoid unnecessary tissue plane violation.

Creating a Working Space

Retro-auricular approach is an open surgery. No gas insufflation is involved. The incision is taken behind the ear lobule, initially cranially and then turned posteriorly at the level of the external auditory canal, and then horizontally up to 5 mm inside the hairline. The incision is then turned inferiorly and posteriorly, staying 5 mm inside the hairline up to about 5–6 cm. The skin flaps are raised at a subplatysmal plane, staying over the sternomastoid muscle, preserving a layer of fascia over the

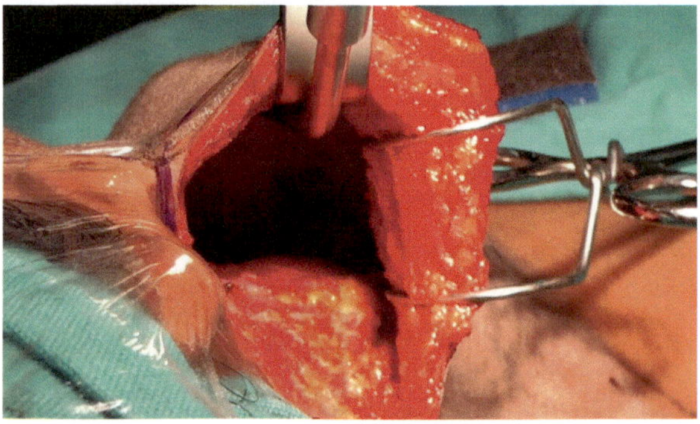

Fig. 10.6 Retro-auricular, working space after elevation

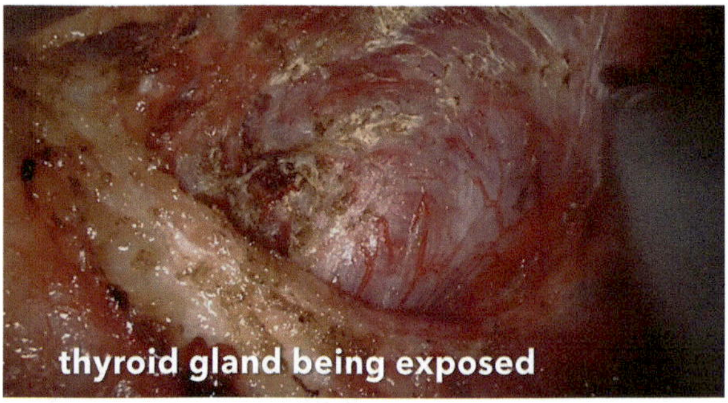

Fig. 10.7 Retro-auricular, thyroid gland exposure

muscle. Injury to the great auricular nerve and the external jugular vein is to be avoided. The dissection is then proceeded inferiorly to reach the suprasternal notch in the midline and the clavicular level laterally. Too much lateral dissection is not necessary for a thyroidectomy without neck dissection. The flap may have to be raised past the midline. After the working space is created (Fig. 10.5), the self-retaining retractor is introduced and placed to maintain the height of the space for robotic docking (Fig. 10.6).

Docking stage

The robot is docked. A 30° scope is used face down and placed centrally along the blade of the retractor. The authors place the scope in the second or the third arm on the Xi system. The Maryland forceps is held to the left of the scope and curved monopolar scissors to the right. The Prograsp forceps is placed on the remaining extreme arm, either 1 or 4, depending on the surgery side.

Console stage (surgical resection of the thyroid gland)

1. The investing layer of the deep cervical fascia is separated initially from the anterior border of the sternomastoid muscle. The Prograsp forceps can hold and retract the tissue, whereas the Maryland forceps and the curved scissors are used to dissect and cut the tissue. All the vessels that are encountered can be coagulated and cut

2. Omohyoid, sternohyoid, and sternothyroid muscles are then sequentially identified, delineated and retracted to visualise the anterior surface of the thyroid (Fig. 10.7), the isthmus, and the inferior border of the gland.
3. Superior pole vessels are dissected and delineated, coagulated, and cut.
4. The dissection proceeds medially, and the external branch of the superior laryngeal nerve is seen entering the cricothyroid muscle. Subsequently, the medial dissection is done to divide the isthmus.
5. Attention is then turned laterally and inferiorly, retracting the superior pole medially. The dissection is maintained close to the capsule of the gland without breaching it. The middle thyroid vein is identified, coagulated, and cut. The inferior thyroid artery is identified, coagulated close to the gland, and cut. The dissection in the loose areolar tissue laterally will identify the recurrent laryngeal nerve entry point. The nerve may be followed and preserved. It is not necessary to dissect the nerve fully.
6. Dissection is further done to release the inferior pole. Finally, the vessels are coagulated and cut to complete the hemithyroidectomy.
7. Contralateral lobectomy can be done through the same side, but it may be prudent to do it through a contralateral postauricular route in the initial few cases.
8. The contralateral superior pole is identified, coagulated, and cut. The lobe is then released from the trachea by medial dissection, preserving the recurrent laryngeal nerve and parathyroids to complete the thyroidectomy.
9. Haemostasis is checked meticulously; suction drains are inserted and taken out behind the hairline.
10. Closure: Surgical wound is irrigated with warm saline, and the Valsalva manoeuver is applied to check for bleeders. The author preferred to place the drain and wound closed in layers.
11. Postoperative care is not grossly different from open thyroidectomy. Calcium levels should be monitored. The suction drain is removed when the drainage falls below 20 mL/day. The patient may be discharged the following day.

10.5.2 Trans-axillary/Breast Approach

Several modifications are described in the literature by several authors using the robot with multiple small port incisions to a single large incision [25]. Here, we discuss three main standard robotic approaches. (1) Axillo-Bilateral-Breast Approach (ABBA), (2) Bilateral-Axillo-Breast-Approach (BABA)—This approach provides a symmetrical view to both lobes of the thyroid and prevents instruments overcrowding. (3) Robot-assisted breast-axillo insufflation thyroidectomy (RABIT) approach is a modification [26]. A summary of the equipment and surgical techniques is given below [25, 27].

10.5.2.1 Surgical Equipment

The main equipment are:

- The da Vinci Si/Xi robot
- The robotic instruments
  - Prograsp forceps
  - Maryland dissector
  - Harmonic scalpel Ethicon
- The 30° endoscope
- Modified Chung retractor
- NIM (nerve integrity monitor) endotracheal tube
- SSEP (Somato Sensory Evoked Potentials)
- Handheld recurrent laryngeal nerve stimulator
- Alexis wound protector/retractor
- Electrocautery with a short, regular and long tip
- Vascular DeBakey
- Army-navy retractors
- Right-angled retractors
- Breast lighted retractors

10.5.2.2 Preparation and Procedure

Patient positioning

Patient neck is slightly extended with a small shoulder bag, and the ipsilateral arm is extended and placed on the patient's head with flexion at the elbow, as described by Ikeda et al., to avoid a stretch on the upper limb nerves.

Skin preparation and incision

An axillary, 8 cm skin incision (Fig. 10.8) is made on the lateral border of the pectoralis major muscle, and skin flap (Fig. 10.9) elevated superficial to this muscle on the chest and in the sub-platysmal plane in the neck.

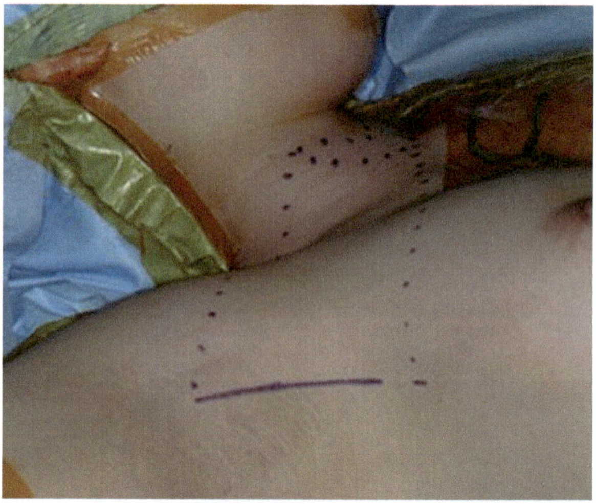

Fig. 10.8 Trans-axillary incision

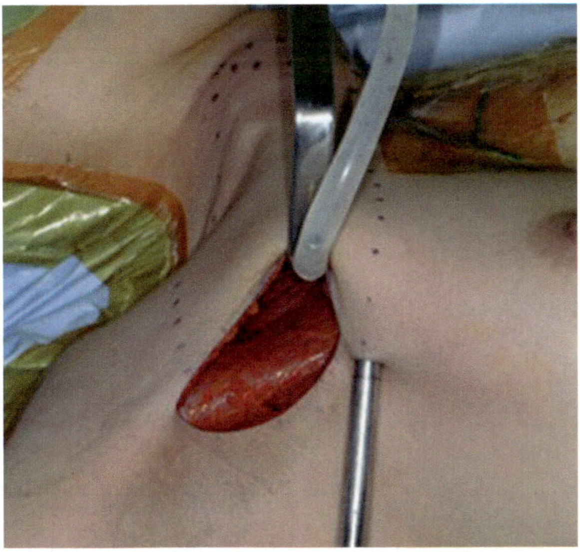

Fig. 10.9 Trans-axillary working space after the flap is raised

Creating a working space

Identifying the sternomastoid insertion is essential, then entering the avascular space between the sternal and clavicular heads of the sternomastoid muscle. Omohyoid muscle is identified, retracted superficially and posterolaterally. Strap muscles are identified and dissected off the thyroid to the lateral border of the contralateral thyroid lobe. Chung retractor is placed and fixed to maintain working space.

Docking stage

Three robotic arms consisting of a camera, Maryland dissector and harmonic scalpel are docked in the working space. The camera is placed in the centre position, dissector and harmonic scalpel placed on either side of the camera without any collision. The fourth robotic arm with Prograsp forceps can be inserted through a 0.8 mm port in the anterior chest wall.

Console stage (surgical resection of the thyroid gland)

The superior pole of the thyroid is grasped with Prograsp forceps and retracted medially, and blunt dissection is done to identify the superior laryngeal nerve's external branch. Superior thyroid vascular pedicle is ligated close to the gland with a harmonic scalpel. The superior parathyroid gland is identified and preserved. Blunt haemostatic is dissection done with the help of Maryland dissector and harmonic scalpel, recurrent laryngeal nerve identified at the entry point into the cricothyroid muscle and preserved. The inferior parathyroid gland is identified and preserved. The thyroid lobe is detached from the berry ligament with sharp dissection and specimen delivered in a plastic bag. RLN integrity is tested and confirmed with the nerve monitor. Robotic arms are retracted from the surgical field. The surgical field (Fig. 10.10) is irrigated with warm saline, and haemostasis is confirmed

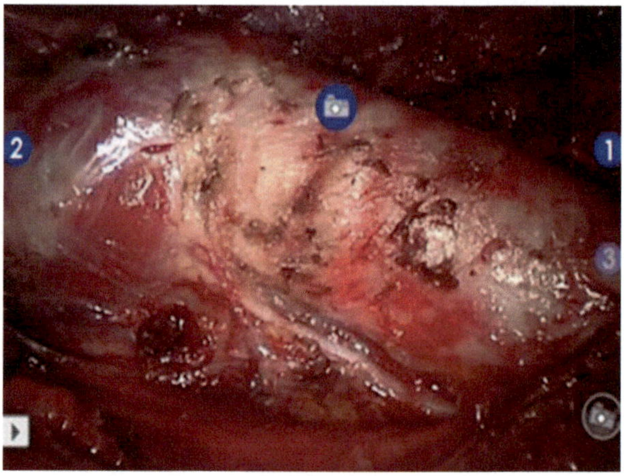

Fig. 10.10 Surgical thyroidectomy bed after a trans-axillary thyroidectomy

with Valsalva manoeuvre. The suction drain would be secured, and the wound closed in layers.

Robot-assisted breast-axillo insufflation thyroidectomy (RABIT) approach [26] is a modification of the robotic BABA approach described by Lee et al. [28]

10.5.3 Robotic trans-oral thyroidectomy

Trans-oral thyroidectomy is becoming popular. A truly scarless approach is the advantage. The operation is done through a median, central approach, allowing bilateral exploration of the thyroid gland and central compartment. Endoscopic approaches [29] and robotic approaches are described [30]. A summary of the robotic approach is given below [30, 31]. An ideal patient for trans-oral thyroidectomy would be:

- Uncomplicated thyroid nodule up to 3 cm
- No obesity, not too short neck
- Females
- Male patient is more challenging (laryngeal prominence/thyroid cartilage is larger in adult men)
- Left lobectomy is more challenging for the right-hand surgeon

10.5.3.1 Preparation and Procedure

Patient positioning
Patient is in supine position with neck extended using a sandbag under the shoulder.

Oral mucosal incision
Three incisions are made. The first one is a midline incision, about 2 cm from the frenulum in a horizontal fashion (Fig. 10.11). The other two (Fig. 10.12) are on either side on the mucosal aspect of the angle of the mouth.

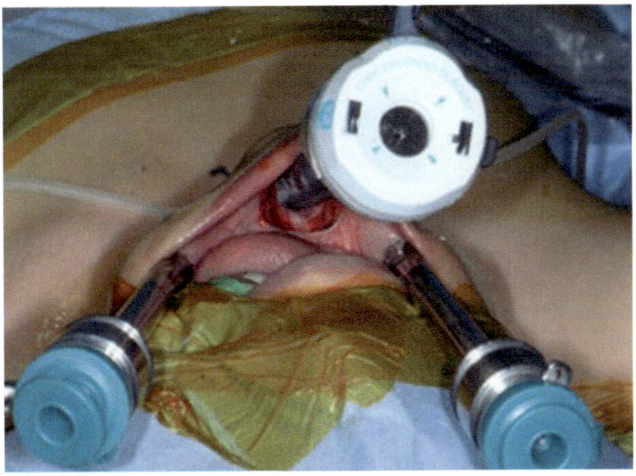

Fig. 10.11 Trans-oral midline incision

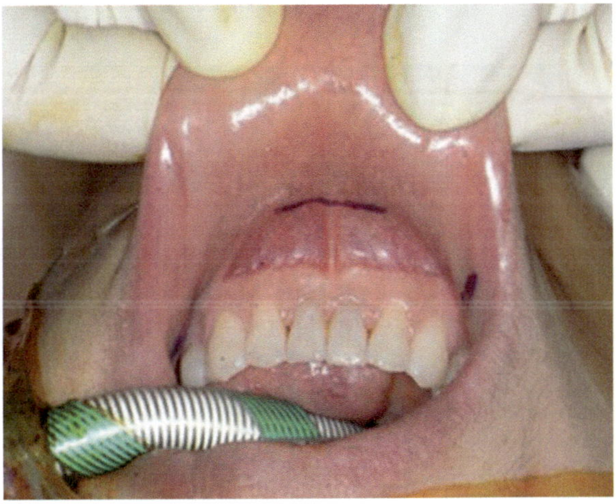

Fig. 10.12 Trans-oral lateral incisions after the ports are introduced

Creating a working space

A sub-platysmal flap is intended to be created using the three incisions. First, the midline incision is addressed using a blunt dissection technique to reach the lower border of the mandible. Following this, a sub-platysmal flap is raised in the midline over the strap muscles up to the supra-sternal notch. This may be facilitated by infiltration of normal saline mixed with adrenaline. A 30° endoscope is introduced through this, and carbon-di-oxide insufflation at 8–10 L/min is done through this port. Similarly, sub-platysmal dissection is done through the other two incisions as well.

Docking stage

The robotic system is deployed (Fig. 10.13). The cannulae are then introduced. The central cannula is used to secure the endoscope. This is followed by the Maryland dissector and Harmonic scalpel through the right and left angle of mouth ports, respectively.

Fig. 10.13 Trans-oral docking

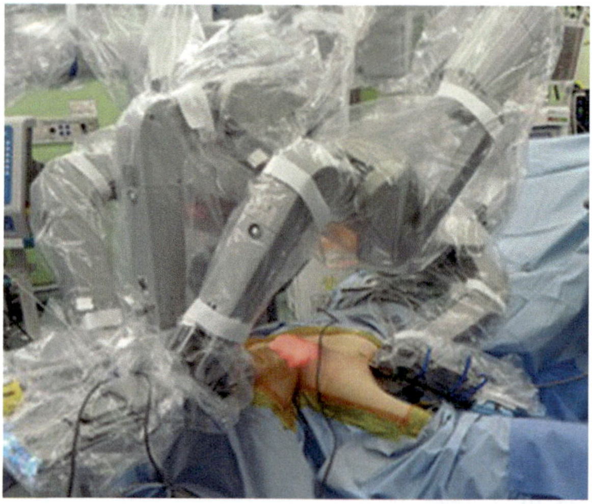

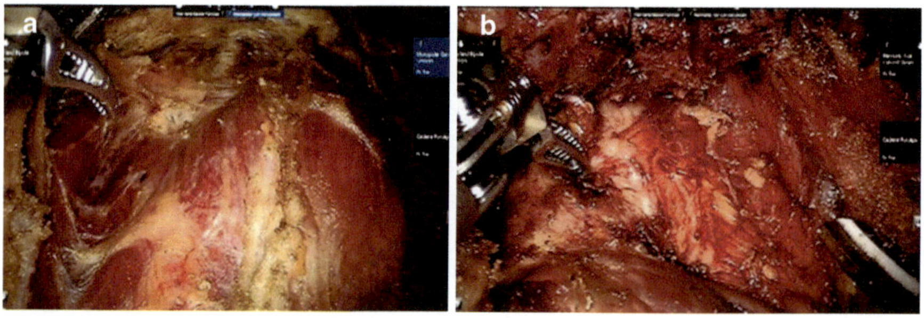

Fig. 10.14 (**a**) Trans-oral thyroidectomy, midline and the straps are being separated; (**b**) Trans-oral thyroidectomy bed after surgery

Console stage (surgical resection of the thyroid gland)

The dissection begins in the mid-line (Fig. 10.14a). The strap muscles are separated and then elevated off the thyroid gland to expose the thyroid lobe being addressed first. The pyramidal lobe is identified and dissected of the thyroid cartilage. Isthmectomy is performed to free the thyroid lobe from the trachea in the midline. Following this, the superior pole is identified, and each vessel is ligated individually. The superior parathyroid gland is identified and preserved. The superior pole is retracted inferiorly, and the recurrent-laryngeal nerve is identified at its point of entry into the larynx. The thyroid is dissected off the Berry's ligament. The inferior dissection is then continued, and the inferior parathyroid gland is identified and preserved. Hemi thyroidectomy is thus completed (Fig. 10.14b). The procedure is repeated on the opposite side when indicated.

10.6 Complications and Outcomes: A Comparison with Open Thyroidectomy

10.6.1 Postoperative Pain

Post-operative pain in the immediate period and chronic pain over 3–6 months have been studied. Overall evidence suggested that RT and OT were comparable for post-operative pain and the requirement of analgesics. There is extensive flap elevation in most of the approaches of RT; however, the retro-auricular approach reduces it by 38% [32, 33].

10.6.2 Recurrent Laryngeal Nerve Injury

In literature, there is no universal definition of transient and permanent RLN palsy. However, their incidences in RT vary between 1 and 7% for transient injury and 0–2% for permanent injury. This is comparable with OT [32, 34–36].

10.6.3 Brachial Plexus Injury

The potential of a brachial plexus injury is a complication of the trans-axillary RT, which is not encountered in a usual thyroidectomy. Although it has a low incidence of 0.2%, it is a debilitating and worrying complication for the patient. This can be avoided by other approaches [37].

10.6.4 Hypoparathyroidism

The definitions of postoperative, transient and permanent hypoparathyroidism differed among various studies. However, all available meta-analyses showed that the current risk of transient and permanent hypothyroidism is not increased with RT. The reported rates of transient and permanent hypoparathyroidism in RT ranged from 0–53% and 0–3%, respectively [32, 35, 36, 38, 39].

10.6.5 Bleeding and Hematoma

These are known life-threatening complications of thyroidectomy. An incidence of 2–3% has been reported in patients undergoing RT, which is comparable with OT [32, 35, 36, 38, 39].

10.6.6 Voice and Swallowing Function

The patient's voice, irrespective of the RLN function status, has been studied, and short-term and long-term outcomes suggest better results with RT than OT [32, 40]. Similar comparatively better outcomes have been noted in swallowing function post RT.

10.6.7 Paraesthesia

Significantly higher chest and neck paraesthesia has been reported in RT due to more extensive skin flap elevation. However, these sensations over the chest wall skin are regained considerably after 3 months of surgery. Retroauricular thyroidectomy can result in an altered sensation of the pinna and behind the ear. Hypertrophic scar in the post-auricular area is also common [32, 41].

10.6.8 Cosmetic Satisfaction

Cosmetic advantage is the most important outcome of RT and gains superiority over OT in all studies. The degree of psychological distress is also shown to have reduced with RT. [42]

10.6.9 Complications Specific to Trans-Oral Approaches

Mental nerve injury, skin burns, temporary chin numbness and oral commissure tears. Neck infections can also rarely occur.

10.7 Economic Parameters

10.7.1 Peri-Operative Time

Liu et al. [43], in an evidence-based review of 19 comparative studies and seven meta-analyses, showed that the operating time for robotic thyroidectomy is significantly more than that of open thyroidectomy. But, on comparing robotic and endoscopic thyroidectomy, Lang et al. found no significant difference in the total operating time when a robot was used. Considering the extra steps of surgery involved in RT compared to OT, in the form of docking and elevation of the skin flaps, it may hardly be ever possible to compare the time taken in RT to that of OT. However, with the increased experience, the time taken for RT ought to reduce.

10.7.2 Hospital Stay

The total duration of hospital stay is the same for robotic and open thyroidectomy. However, there is an increasing trend to promote thyroidectomy as a day case procedure [32, 38, 43].

10.7.3 Cost

The robotic setup is expensive, and the cost gets added to the surgical cost. Duration of surgery and operation theatre time also is an added disadvantage when the cost is concerned. The cost includes the initial establishment cost, the maintenance cost and the cost of instruments and disposables. The instruments have a cap on the number of surgeries they can be used. The cost of RT is shown to be 2.1 times that of OT [44, 45].

10.8 Oncological Outcomes

Considering RT is not a contra-indication for differentiated thyroid cancer, it is prudent to look at the oncological outcomes [32, 43] of RT compared to OT. Central compartment neck dissection is also being performed contentedly through the robotic approach at the same time when indicated. The oncological outcomes can be studied as lymph node retrieval, surgical completeness of resection, tumour recurrence, and survival outcomes. Considering good survival outcomes in general for differentiated thyroid carcinomas compared to other head and neck malignancies, survival outcomes need a long-term follow-up for thyroid cancer. While survival outcomes have not extensively been compared between RT and OT, Lymph node retrieval and completeness of resection have been studied in at least three published meta-analyses [36, 39, 46].

10.8.1 Completeness of Resection

Post thyroidectomy, for differentiated thyroid cancer, the completeness of resection is assessed by radioactive iodine (RAI) uptake on post-therapy whole body scan as well as the thyrotropin (TSH)-stimulated serum thyroglobulin (sTg) level. Two meta-analyses by Wang et al. and Son et al. did not find any difference for stimulated thyroglobulin levels. However, Lang et al., in a meta-analysis including a large number of single studies, showed a considerably high sTg level in RT as compared to OT, indicating towards, like explained, an incompleteness of resection. Evidence suggests that the amount of remnant thyroid tissue as reflected by the sTg level may be higher post RT than post OT. However, this is reported to be resolved after RAI ablation [36, 39, 46].

10.8.2 Lymph Node Retrieval

Radical central compartment dissection is considered the hallmark of oncological control. The number of lymph nodes retrieved in RT is lower than in OT in three meta-analyses. However, the lymph node retrieval for lateral neck dissection is similar in both. RT may be inferior in the number of lymph nodes retrieved from the central compartment [36, 39, 46, 47].

10.8.3 Survival and Recurrence

Short-term locoregional recurrence within the first two postoperative years is comparable between RT and OT. In the only long-term follow-up study by Lee et al., the rates of locoregional recurrence at 5 years was 1.2% for both RT and OT. The survival outcomes between RT and OT were compared, and at 5-year follow-up, no significant difference between RT and OT for the disease-free survival was observed (99.7% versus 98.7%, $P = 0.89$). Considering the good survival outcomes of DTC, a longer time may be needed to compare survival outcomes and recurrences between robotic and open thyroidectomy [47, 48].

10.9 Advantages of Robotic Thyroidectomy

The advantages [24] of robotic thyroidectomy are:

10.9.1 Visualisation

RT allows a three-dimensional view. A tenfold greater magnification and high definition are achieved as compared to the human eye. The vision is surgeon controlled and, unlike endoscopic thyroidectomy, does not need an assistant to hold the camera.

10.9.2 Dexterity

An enhanced dexterity due to the wristed hand movements is possible. Seven degrees of freedom on movements have been described, shoulder roll, wrist yaw, arm yaw, wrist roll, wrist pinch, shoulder pinch, and elbow pinch.

10.9.3 Retraction

The fourth arm of the robot helps in retraction. A bedside assistant also helps with suctioning and retraction. This helps in further better visualisation during surgery.

10.9.4 Precision

The robot neutralises surgeon tremor: the enhanced visualisation, abled dexterity and stable retraction help precision in surgery. Thus, reducing surgical complications such as nerve damage and parathyroid ischemia.

10.9.5 Surgeon Ergonomics

The operating surgeon can comfortably sit in the robot console once the docking is complete.

10.10 Limitations of Robotic Thyroidectomy

The limitations of robotic thyroidectomy are: [24]

10.10.1 Cost

It includes the initial establishment cost, annual maintenance cost, disposable instruments cost. The cost involved in the prolonged anaesthesia and operative time may also contribute. The cost can be reduced by multidisciplinary use, especially in an institutional practice.

10.10.2 Learning curve

An initial adequate pre-clinical training is essential. Basic instrumental training is received on animal and human cadavers. A learning of 30–40 cases is reported for robotic thyroidectomy. A proper case selection is during this learning curve. It is ideal that the initial few cases are done with guidance and proctoring from an experienced peer.

10.10.3 Lack of haptic feedback

The absence of haptic feedback may initially be difficult as one must rely on visual clues to assess the surgical field. This can lead to crushing of tissues and inadvertent injury to the vital structures.

10.10.4 Operative time

Considering the extra steps of surgery involved in RT compared to OT, in the form of docking and elevation of the skin flaps, it may hardly be ever possible to compare the time taken in RT to that of OT. However, with the increased experience, the time taken for RT ought to reduce.

10.11 Latest Advances and Future

Single port robotic thyroidectomy is now being done in many centres across South Korea. Retro-auricular, trans-axillary and trans-oral approaches using the single port system is reported [49–51]. The present robotic system has many limitations as mentioned above. Innovative technology with newer robots are under different stages of development. They may be launched soon. Future surgical robots may be flexible and smaller. They might also incorporate intraoperative neuro-monitoring, non-optical viewing, haptic feedback, and a navigation system for the parathyroid glands, recurrent laryngeal nerve, and lymph nodes. Such innovative surgical robots may make robotic thyroidectomy safer and more effective, and minimally invasive [52]. Remote site surgeries may be possible.

10.12 Conclusions

Robotic-assisted thyroidectomy surgery is a safe procedure for carefully selected patients with a benign or malignant thyroid mass. It avoids a neck scar with various added advantages of surgical precision from using a robot. Remote access approaches use well-hidden incisions. They are not minimally invasive. Robotic approaches score above endoscopic methods. Robotic approaches are feasible, safe and cosmetically better. Though long-term follow-up is lacking, there are many reports using it for malignant thyroid tumours. Patient selection is important. Sufficient cadaver and preclinical training should be undertaken. Standardised and formal teaching for robotic surgical skills is necessary. Continued accumulation of evidence regarding technical and oncological safety is vital. The long learning curve and cost are the limitations. However, worldwide there have been a more positive trend and rising popularity towards robotic thyroidectomy.

Acknowledgement The authors acknowledge Prof Kyung Tae, Professor, Department of Otolaryngology-Head and Neck Surgery College of Medicine, Hanyang University, Seoul, Korea, for the Figures 10.8–10.14.

References

1. Vander JB, Gaston EA, Dawber TR. The significance of nontoxic thyroidnodules. Final report of a 15-year study of the incidence of thyroid malignancy. Ann Intern Med. 1968;69(3):537–40.
2. Hüscher CS, Chiodini S, Napolitano C, Recher A. Endoscopic right thyroid lobectomy. Surg Endosc. 1997;11(8):877. https://doi.org/10.1007/s004649900476.
3. Chung WY. The evolution of robotic thyroidectomy: from inception to neck dissection. J Robot Surg. 2011;5:17–23. https://doi.org/10.1007/s11701-010-0232-9.
4. Gagner M. Endoscopic subtotal parathyroidectomy in patients with primary hyperparathyroidism. Br J Surg. 1996;83(6):875. https://doi.org/10.1002/bjs.1800830656.
5. Miccoli P, Bellantone R, Mourad M, Walz M, Raffaelli M, Berti P. Minimally invasive video-assisted thyroidectomy: multiinstitutional experience. World J Surg. 2002;26(8):972–5. https://doi.org/10.1007/s00268-002-6627-7. Epub 2002 May 21.
6. Ohgami M, Ishii S, Arisawa Y, Ohmori T, Noga K, Furukawa T, Kitajima M. Scarless endoscopic thyroidectomy: breast approach for better cosmesis. Surg Laparosc Endosc Percutan Tech. 2000;10(1):1–4.
7. Ikeda Y, Takami H, Niimi M, Kan S, Sasaki Y, Takayama J. Endoscopic thyroidectomy by the axillary approach. Surg Endosc. 2001;15(11):1362–4. https://doi.org/10.1007/s004640080139. Epub 2001 Aug 16.
8. Shimazu K, Shiba E, Tamaki Y, Takiguchi S, Taniguchi E, Ohashi S, Noguchi S. Endoscopic thyroid surgery through the axillo-bilateral-breast approach. Surg Laparosc Endosc Percutan Tech. 2003;13(3):196–201. https://doi.org/10.1097/00129689-200306000-00011.
9. Bärlehner E, Benhidjeb T. Cervical scarless endoscopic thyroidectomy: axillo-bilateral-breast approach (ABBA). Surg Endosc. 2008;22(1):154–7. https://doi.org/10.1007/s00464-007-9393-7. Epub 2007 Apr 13.
10. Choe JH, Kim SW, Chung KW, Park KS, Han W, Noh DY, Oh SK, Youn YK. Endoscopic thyroidectomy using a new bilateral axillo-breast approach. World J Surg. 2007;31(3):601–6. https://doi.org/10.1007/s00268-006-0481-y.
11. Lee KE, Kim HY, Park WS, Choe JH, Kwon MR, Oh SK, Youn YK. Postauricular and axillary approach endoscopic neck surgery: a new technique. World J Surg. 2009;33(4):767–72. https://doi.org/10.1007/s00268-009-9922-8.
12. Wilhelm T, Harlaar JJ, Kerver A, Kleinrensink GJ, Benhidjeb T. Surgical anatomy of the floor of the oral cavity and the cervical spaces as a rationale for trans-oral, minimal-invasive endoscopic surgical procedures: results of anatomical studies. Eur Arch Otorrinolaringol. 2010;267(8):1285–90. https://doi.org/10.1007/s00405-010-1219-x. Epub 2010 Feb 24.
13. Wilhelm T, Metzig A. Video. Endoscopic minimally invasive thyroidectomy: first clinical experience. Surg Endosc. 2010;24(7):1757–8. https://doi.org/10.1007/s00464-009-0820-9. Epub 2009 Dec 25.
14. Nakajo A, Arima H, Hirata M, Mizoguchi T, Kijima Y, Mori S, Ishigami S, Ueno S, Yoshinaka H, Natsugoe S. Trans-Oral Video-Assisted Neck Surgery (TOVANS). A new transoral technique of endoscopic thyroidectomy with gasless premandible approach. Surg Endosc. 2013;27(4):1105–10. https://doi.org/10.1007/s00464-012-2588-6. Epub 2012 Nov 21.
15. Richmon JD, Holsinger FC, Kandil E, Moore MW, Garcia JA, Tufano RP. Transoral robotic-assisted thyroidectomy with central neck dissection: preclinical cadaver feasibility study and proposed surgical technique. J Robot Surg. 2011;5(4):279–82. https://doi.org/10.1007/s11701-011-0287-2. Epub 2011 Jun 15.
16. Park JO, Kim CS, Song JN, Kim JE, Nam IC, Lee SY, Chun BJ, Cho JH, Joo YH, Cho KJ, Park YH, Kim MS, Sun DI. Transoral endoscopic thyroidectomy via the tri-vestibular routes: results of a preclinical cadaver feasibility study. Eur Arch Otorrinolaringol. 2014;271(12):3269–75. https://doi.org/10.1007/s00405-014-2911-z. Epub 2014 Feb 5.

17. Park JO, Sun DI. Transoral endoscopic thyroidectomy: our initial experience using a new endoscopic technique. Surg Endosc. 2017;31(12):5436–43. https://doi.org/10.1007/s00464-017-5594-x. Epub 2017 May 18.
18. Kang SW, Jeong JJ, Yun JS, Sung TY, Lee SC, Lee YS, Nam KH, Chang HS, Chung WY, Park CS. Robot-assisted endoscopic surgery for thyroid cancer: experience with the first 100 patients. Surg Endosc. 2009;23(11):2399–406. https://doi.org/10.1007/s00464-009-0366-x. Epub 2009 Mar 5.
19. Walvekar RR, Wallace E, Bergeron B, Whitworth R, Beahm DD, Nuss DW. Retro-auricular video-assisted "gasless" thyroidectomy: feasibility study in human cadavers. Surg Endosc. 2010;24(11):2895–9. https://doi.org/10.1007/s00464-010-1068-0. Epub 2010 Apr 24.
20. Terris DJ, Singer MC, Seybt MW. Robotic facelift thyroidectomy: II. Clinical feasibility and safety. Laryngoscope. 2011;121(8):1636–41. https://doi.org/10.1002/lary.21832. Epub 2011 Jun 30.
21. Lee HY, You JY, Woo SU, Son GS, Lee JB, Bae JW, Kim HY. Transoral periosteal thyroidectomy: cadaver to human. Surg Endosc. 2015;29(4):898–904. https://doi.org/10.1007/s00464-014-3749-6. Epub 2014 Aug 15.
22. Thankappan K, Iyer S. Initiating a robotic thyroidectomy program in India. Indian J Surg Oncol. 2018;9(2):241–6. https://doi.org/10.1007/s13193-018-0746-6.
23. Berber E, Bernet V, Fahey TJ 3rd, Kebebew E, Shaha A, Stack BC Jr, Stang M, Steward DL, Terris DJ, American Thyroid Association Surgical Affairs Committee. American Thyroid Association statement on remote-access thyroid surgery. Thyroid. 2016;26(3):331–7. https://doi.org/10.1089/thy.2015.0407.
24. Thankappan K. Robotic retro-auricular thyroidectomy: indications and technique. J Head Neck Phys Surg. 2019;7:6–10.
25. Chang EHE, Kim HY, Koh YW, Chung WY. Overview of robotic thyroidectomy. Gland Surg. 2017;6(3):218–28. https://doi.org/10.21037/gs.2017.03.18.
26. Nayak SP, Sadhoo A, Gangadhara B, Reddy S, Khan A, Munisiddaiah D, Ramakrishnan A. Robotic-assisted breast-axillo insufflation thyroidectomy (RABIT): a retrospective case series of thyroid carcinoma. Int J Clin Oncol. 2020;25(3):439–45.
27. Bhatia P, Mohamed HE, Kadi A, Kandil E, Walvekar RR. Remote access thyroid surgery. Gland Surg. 2015;4(5):376–87. https://doi.org/10.3978/j.issn.2227-684X.2015.05.02.
28. Lee KE, Choi JY, Youn Y-K. Bilateral axillo-breast approach robotic thyroidectomy. Surg Laparosc Endosc Percutan Tech. 2011;21:230–6. https://doi.org/10.1097/SLE.0b013e31822d045.
29. Dionigi G, Lavazza M, Wu CW, Sun H, Liu X, Tufano RP, Kim HY, Richmon JD, Anuwong A. Transoral thyroidectomy: why is it needed? Gland Surg. 2017;6(3):272–6. https://doi.org/10.21037/gs.2017.03.21.
30. Tae K, Ji YB, Song CM, Park JS, Park JH, Kim DS. Safety and efficacy of transoral robotic and endoscopic thyroidectomy: the first 100 cases. Head Neck. 2020;42(2):321–9. https://doi.org/10.1002/hed.25999.
31. Richmon JD, Kim HY. Transoral robotic thyroidectomy (TORT): procedures and outcomes. Gland Surg. 2017;6(3):285–9. https://doi.org/10.21037/gs.2017.05.05.
32. Lee IS, Kwon EH, Bae, Chung WY. Comparative analysis of oncological outcomes and quality of life after robotic versus conventional open thyroidectomy with modified radical neck dissection in patients with papillary thyroid carcinoma and lateral neck node metastases. J Clin Endocrinol Metab. 2013;98(7):2701–8.
33. Ryu HR, Lee J, Park J-H, et al. A comparison of postoperative pain after conventional open thyroidectomy and transaxillary single-incision robotic thyroidectomy: a prospective study. Ann Surg Oncol. 2013;20(7):2279–84.
34. Kandil E, Hammad AY, Walvekar RR, Hu T, Masoodi H, Mohamed SE, Deniwar A, Stack BC Jr. Robotic thyroidectomy versus nonrobotic approaches: a meta-analysis examining surgical outcomes. Surg Innov. 2016;23(3):317–25. https://doi.org/10.1177/1553350615613451. Epub 2015 Nov 2.

35. Jackson NR, Yao L, Tufano RP, Kandil EH. Safety of robotic thyroidectomy approaches: meta-analysis and systematic review. Head Neck. 2014;36(1):137–43. https://doi.org/10.1002/hed.23223. Epub 2013 Mar 8.
36. Lang BH, Wong CK, Tsang JS, Wong KP, Wan KY. A systematic review and meta-analysis comparing surgically-related complications between robotic-assisted thyroidectomy and conventional open thyroidectomy. Ann Surg Oncol. 2014;21(3):850–61. https://doi.org/10.1245/s10434-013-3406-7. Epub 2013 Nov 23.
37. Luginbuhl A, et al. Detection of evolving injury to the brachial plexus during transaxillary robotic thyroidectomy. Laryngoscope. 2012;122:110–5.
38. Sun GH, Peress L, Pynnonen MA. Systematic review and meta-analysis of robotic vs conventional thyroidectomy approaches for thyroid disease. Otolaryngol Head Neck Surg. 2014;150(4):520–32. https://doi.org/10.1177/0194599814521779. Epub 2014 Feb 5.
39. Son SK, Kim JH, Bae JS, Lee SH. Surgical safety and oncologic effectiveness in robotic versus conventional open thyroidectomy in thyroid cancer: a systematic review and meta-analysis. Ann Surg Oncol. 2015;22(9):3022–32. https://doi.org/10.1245/s10434-015-4375-9. Epub 2015 Jan 30.
40. Tae K, Kim KY, Yun BR, et al. Functional voice and swallowing outcomes after robotic thyroidectomy by a gasless unilateral axillo-breast approach: comparison with open thyroidectomy. Surg Endosc Other Interv Tech. 2012;26(7):1871–7.
41. Song CM, Ji YB, Bang HS, Park CW, Kim H, Tae K. Long-term sensory disturbance and discomfort after robotic thyroidectomy. World J Surg. 2014;38(7):1743–8.
42. do Koo H, da Kim M, Choi JY, Lee KE, Cho SH, Youn YK. In-depth survey of scarring and distress in patients undergoing bilateral axillo-breast approach robotic thyroidectomy or conventional open thyroidectomy. Surg Laparosc Endosc Percutan Tech. 2015;25(5):436–9.
43. Liu SY, Ng EK. Robotic versus open thyroidectomy for differentiated thyroid cancer: an evidence-based review. Int J Endocrinol. 2016;2016:4309087. https://doi.org/10.1155/2016/4309087. Epub 2016 Mar 16.
44. Cabot JC, Lee CR, Brunaud L, Kleiman DA, Chung WY, Fahey TJ 3rd, Zarnegar R. Robotic and endoscopic transaxillary thyroidectomies may be cost prohibitive when compared to standard cervical thyroidectomy: a cost analysis. Surgery. 2012;152(6):1016–24. https://doi.org/10.1016/j.surg.2012.08.029.
45. Broome JT, Pomeroy S, Solorzano CC. Expense of robotic thyroidectomy: a cost analysis at a single institution. Arch Surg. 2012;147(12):1102–6. https://doi.org/10.1001/archsurg.2012.1870.
46. Wang YC, Liu K, Xiong JJ, Zhu JQ. Robotic thyroidectomy versus conventional open thyroidectomy for differentiated thyroid cancer: meta-analysis. J Laryngol Otol. 2015;129(6):558–67. https://doi.org/10.1017/S002221511500122X.
47. Kang SW, Lee SH, Park JH, Jeong JS, Park S, Lee CR, Jeong JJ, Nam KH, Chung WY, Park CS. A comparative study of the surgical outcomes of robotic and conventional open modified radical neck dissection for papillary thyroid carcinoma with lateral neck node metastasis. Surg Endosc. 2012;26(11):3251–7. https://doi.org/10.1007/s00464-012-2333-1.
48. Lee SG, Lee J, Kim MJ, Choi JB, Kim TH, Ban EJ, Lee CR, Kang SW, Jeong JJ, Nam KH, Jo YS, Chung WY. Long-term oncologic outcome of robotic versus open total thyroidectomy in PTC: a case-matched retrospective study. Surg Endosc. 2016;30(8):3474–9.
49. Noel JE, Lee MC, Tam K, Lim GC, Holsinger FC, Koh YW. Retroauricular thyroidectomy with a single-arm robotic surgical system: preclinical cadaveric study. Head Neck. 2020;42(12):3663–9. https://doi.org/10.1002/hed.26436.
50. Kim K, Kang SW, Kim JK, Lee CR, Lee J, Jeong JJ, Nam KH, Chung WY. Robotic transaxillary hemithyroidectomy using the da Vinci SP robotic system: initial experience with 10 consecutive cases. Surg Innov. 2020;27(3):256–64. https://doi.org/10.1177/1553350620909279.
51. Tae K. Transoral robotic thyroidectomy using the da Vinci single-port surgical system. Gland Surg. 2020;9(3):614–6. https://doi.org/10.21037/gs.2020.03.37.
52. Tae K, Ji YB, Song CM, Ryu J. Robotic and endoscopic thyroid Surgery: evolution and advances. Clin Exp Otorhinolaryngol. 2019;12(1):1–11. https://doi.org/10.21053/ceo.2018.00766.

Complications of Thyroid Surgery (Except Vocal Cord Palsy)

11

P. V. Pradeep

11.1 Introduction

Like any surgical procedure, thyroid surgery also has complications that can be related to the surgery or could be due to the co-morbidities present in a particular patient. It also depends on the expertise of the surgeon and his team in these kinds of surgeries.

Complications specific to thyroid surgery can generally be divided into major and minor ones. The major complications are those which need immediate intervention or can produce significant morbidity. These include hematoma, stridor, hypocalcaemic tetany, thyrotoxic storm, tracheomalacia. The minor complications are ones that are not life-threatening and do not produce long-lasting morbidity. This included flap oedema, seroma, unilateral vocal cord palsy, superior laryngeal nerve injury, biochemical hypocalcaemia, wound infection, Horner's syndrome, chyle leak, keloid, etc. In the long term, poorly controlled post thyroidectomy hypothyroidism and recurrence can affect the quality of life.

11.2 Hypocalcaemia

The reported incidence of hypocalcaemia varies widely (1–50%) [1–3]. It can be temporary or permanent. It is said to be permanent if hypocalcaemia lasts for more than 6 months. It can be symptomatic hypocalcaemia or biochemical hypocalcaemia. Hypocalcaemia can be influenced by factors such as vitamin D deficiency, hyperthyroidism, and pre-existing calcium deficiency prior to the surgery as in malabsorption states.

P. V. Pradeep (✉)
Department of Endocrine Surgery, Baby Memorial Hospital, Kozhikode, Kerala, India

C. G. Nair, S. J. Abraham (eds.), *Surgical Management of Thyroid and Parathyroid Diseases*, https://doi.org/10.1007/978-981-97-3774-1_11

Further, it is influenced by intraoperative factors. These include whether the parathyroids were identified and protected with intact vascularity, how many parathyroids were saved without devascularisation, and whether any parathyroids were auto-transplanted. Auto-transplanted parathyroids take 2–3 weeks to become active.

Prevention of parathyroid devascularisation is achieved by meticulous dissection, refraining from applying suction/cautery near the gland, and avoiding ligature of the inferior thyroid artery trunk. Only peripheral terminal branches of the inferior thyroid artery are ligated close to the thyroid gland. Even though some authors have recommended preserving at least one full parathyroid gland to prevent permanent hypocalcaemia others feel that at least three parathyroids are necessary to maintain calcium homoeostasis [4]. If there is the possibility of devascularisation of the parathyroid or not possible to preserve it, then it should be auto-transplanted to the sternocleidomastoid muscle in the neck. This approach decreases the incidence of permanent hypoparathyroidism [5, 6]. Intraoperative PTH estimation can help to predict post thyroidectomy hypocalcaemia (PTH <10 pg/mL) [7]. This enables the surgeon to discharge the patients early if there is no risk of developing hypocalcaemia [8].

Symptoms of hypocalcaemia include perioral numbness and paraesthesia which later involve the hands and feet. Later, patients develop carpopedal spasms. Carpal spasms can be spontaneous or can be induced by applying the sphygmomanometer cuff and maintaining cuff pressure 20 mm more than the systolic BP for 2–3 min (Trousseau's sign). Chvostek's sign—twitching of the facial muscles on tapping the facial nerve in front of the tragus is found in hypocalcaemia but is reported to have significant false-positive results.

Biochemical hypocalcaemia needs calcium carbonate supplementation (1–2 g/day). Hypocalcaemia with mild symptoms like numbness/paraesthesia needs calcium supplementation with activated vitamin D (1,25 dihydroxy cholecalciferol). Severe symptoms require intravenous calcium gluconate either as bolus or infusions. Infusion is prepared by adding calcium gluconate ampoules to normal saline and infusing at the rate of 1–2 mg/kg/h. The infusion is tapered over 24–48 h depending on the improvement of symptoms. Once stabilised they are supplemented with oral calcium and vitamin D [9].

Permanent hypocalcaemia is a major concern since it is associated with significant impairment of quality of life, development of cataracts, basal ganglia calcifications, and changes in bone metabolism.

11.2.1 Injury to the Superior Laryngeal Nerve

This complication is less reported since it is difficult to assess. Laryngeal electromyography is needed to make a diagnosis [10]. The superior laryngeal nerve which arises from the vagus divides at the level of hyoid bone into external and internal branches. The external branch (EBSLN) supplies the cricothyroid muscle and has a downward course along the superior thyroid artery before entering the cricothyroid muscle [11]. The relationship of the EBSLN with the superior thyroid artery has been described by Cernea et al. [12]. Cernea Type 2a and 2b are at high risk for injury during thyroid surgery. In order to avoid injury to the external branch, the superior thyroid artery branches are ligated individually and close to the superior pole of the thyroid. Large goitres can significantly alter the position of the EBSLN predisposing it to injury [8]. Apart from preserving the EBSLN, injury to the cricothyroid muscle with blunt dissection or cautery should be avoided. The cricothyroid muscle is tensor of the vocal cord, injury o which results in inability to perform high pitch phonation.

11.3 Haemorrhage and Hematoma

The reported incidence is about 0.1–1.5% [13–15]. There are no specific predisposing factors to this complication in elective thyroid surgery. High surgical volume does not reduce the incidence of hematoma. Careful haemostasis is the most important determinant of this complication. Routine use of neck drain does not prevent postoperative cervical bleeding. The drains can get blocked during an episode of bleeding leading to a hematoma in the neck. Performing the Valsalva manoeuver at the end of the surgery can detect bleeding vessels since this raises the intrapulmonary pressure to 40 cm H_2O.

The manifestations of thyroid bed bleeding will include excessive drain, swelling in the neck, pain in the neck, discomfort in the neck, and if neglected large hematomas can produce tracheal compression and respiratory distress. Most of the bleeding occurs within 6–12 h after thyroidectomy. It has also been reported up to 24 h after the procedure [14]. Timely intervention, neck exploration can save the patient from a catastrophe. Hematoma can also lead to tracheal compression and laryngeal oedema which will make intubation difficult. Hence the surgeon should be ready to open the cervical neck wound and release the hematoma prior to intubation. Tracheostomy is rarely needed in such cases.

11.4 Wound Infection

It is a rare event in thyroidectomy because of the good vasculature. However, immunocompromised patients are susceptible to it. The common organisms are streptococcus or staphylococcus, the incidence being 0.3–0.8% [13, 16]. Antibiotic prophylaxis in immunocompromised individuals is recommended. However, a single dose can be used in normal individuals too. The patient reports redness, oedema over the upper and lower flaps with pain. Fever may or may not be present.

Mild infections without abscess formation need antibiotics like ampicillin and cloxacillin. However, if pus collection is present, it can be drained or aspirated.

11.4.1 Seroma and Flap Oedema

Seromas are seen as boggy swelling at the lower aspect of the wound without and redness of the overlying skin and are mostly painless. Seromas need only aspiration which may have to be repeated under total aseptic precautions. Flap oedema subsides on follow up.

11.4.2 Laryngotracheal Oedema

This can cause respiratory obstruction/stridor. It is rare and can occur after bilateral lymphadenectomy. Disturbances of lymphatic flow cause oedema. It can also occur due to endotracheal intubation and or anaphylactoid reaction [17]. This can be managed with steroids alone or in combination with temporary intubation.

11.4.3 Rare Neural and Vascular Complications

The cervical sympathetic trunk can be injured during operations for retro-oesophageal goitres, locally invasive thyroid cancers. This results in enophthalmos, constricted pupils, and ptosis [1]. The phrenic nerve, the spinal accessory nerve can be injured during neck dissections leading to diaphragmatic palsy and dropping of the shoulder respectively. Pneumothorax has been reported after lymph node dissection at the upper thoracic aperture. Carotid artery injury can happen due to traction or while dissecting thyroid adherent to the artery. Arteriovenous fistula at the upper pole can be prevented by separate ligation of the artery and vein.

11.5 Oesophageal Injury

This can occur in thyroid cancer surgery while dissecting retro-tracheal/retro oesophageal goitres. It is important that such an injury is recognised so that the defect is primarily closed without tension and the patient is kept on nasogastric tube feed or on total parenteral nutrition (TPN). On the 5th postoperative day contrast study can be done to check for leak. If the leak is detected post operatively then the area is drained and TPN/feeding jejunostomy is done till healing occurs.

11.5.1 Thoracic Duct Injury

It is a rare but potentially grave complication after neck surgery. It is likely to occur during neck dissection on the left side. The incidence varies between 1 to 3%. While dissecting the left LJV in its lower part at the root of the neck care is taken to avoid injury to the terminal portion of the thoracic duct. There are reports of chyle leak from the right side also if the right lymphatic duct is injured. A chyle leak is also reported following central compartment neck dissection. If the injury is recognised intraoperatively care is taken to ligate it and drain the area. Cyanoacrylate/fibrin glue can be instilled locally to aid further leak. If detected after surgery prolong milky drain is noticed [18]. The leak is said to be high output if the leak is more than 500 mL/day.

Most of these low output chyle leaks can be managed conservatively with diet modification (low fat, high carbohydrate, and high protein diet) or TPN. Medium-chain triglycerides (MCT) are used in supplements. Octreotide and etilefrine have